The Complete
University Medical Diet

The Complete University Medical Diet

MARIA SIMONSON, Ph.D., Sc.D.

DIRECTOR, HEALTH, WEIGHT AND STRESS
PROGRAM AT JOHNS HOPKINS

AND JOAN RATTNER HEILMAN

Rawson Associates · NEW YORK

Library of Congress Cataloging in Publication Data

Simonson, Maria.
  The complete university medical diet.

  Includes index.
  1. Reducing diets. 2. Reducing—Psychological aspects.
3. Obesity—Psychological aspects. 4. Group therapy.
5. Reducing diets—Recipes. I. Heilman, Joan Rattner.
II. Health, Weight, and Stress Program at Johns Hopkins.
III. Title. [DNLM: 1. Diet, Reducing. WD 210 S611c]
RM222.2.S554 1983   613.2′5   82–42697
ISBN 0–89256–225–0

Published simultaneously in Canada by McClelland and Stewart, Ltd.
Composition by American–Stratford Graphic Services, Inc.
Printed and bound by Fairfield Graphics, Fairfield, Pennsylvania
Designed by Jacques Chazaud
First Edition

To Peggy and Paul Renoff,
whose unflagging enthusiasm, encouragement,
generosity and support for the
Health, Weight and Stress Program at Johns Hopkins
made good health and a happy future
possible for so many.

To my husband,
Gorden,
for his patience, love and encouragement—
for the long hours
dedicated to this program.

Oh would some power the giftie give us
To see ourselves as others see us!

ROBERT BURNS

Todo es posible en esta vida.
Old Spanish Proverb

Contents

AUTHOR'S NOTE

This book is about the Health, Weight and Stress Program which the author originated and has supervised at the Johns Hopkins Medical Institutions for the past fifteen years. However, the reader should be aware that the book is not sponsored or endorsed by the Johns Hopkins Medical Institutions or the Johns Hopkins University. The book is solely the author's product and the author takes full responsibility for it.

The identity of all individuals involved in case studies in this book has been thoroughly disguised for reasons of confidentiality. The essential clinical material is factual and certified.

This book has been written for the sensible, intelligent reader with realistic goals. It is the author's belief that this or any other dietary regimen should be embarked upon only with a physician's permission and carried out only under medical supervision.

ACKNOWLEDGMENTS

A great many people deserve recognition and thanks for making this book possible—so many that all names and services cannot be listed. I must ask forgiveness of those who are omitted but not unappreciated. Titles, university and other affiliations also are omitted because of space limitations. Yet they are well known throughout the professional world.

To all my colleagues and peers in the Johns Hopkins Medical Institutions, my deepest appreciation for their shared research, advice, and encouragement throughout the years.

I am indebted to the following teachers and mentors for their wisdom and guidance: Dr. Albert Stunkard and Dr. Frank Bigsby, and to the late Drs. Bacon Chow, W. Horsley Gantt, and Richard Barnes.

Everlasting appreciation to Dr. Joseph N. Parnes, Dr. Howard Parnes, David Minor, D.D., and the Rev. Janet Kreis—dear friends and pillars of strength—for their guidance and assistance to all involved in our program. To Mark Traynor—my thanks.

Of my loyal, dedicated, professional and administrative staff, whose care and concern for our program is a major contribution, thanks to: Gail Katz, John Gerstley, Dorry Bielecki, Brenda Gretzinger, Joan Werbe, Sue Starr, Anne Wood, Henry Golditch, Miki Welsh, Betty Rehmeyer, Wilson Back, Johanna P., Jean Lundy, Dr. Doreen Moreira, Dr. Janet Gailey-Phipps, Brenda Hume (TYJ), Dr. Alan Harris, Dr. Michael Schmitt, to all my other volunteers, and my co-founder Gwen Campbell. A very special thank you to our medical consultant and advisor, Dr. J. Robert Cockrell, and to Marie McLaughlin, for her work in our adolescent clinic.

Special recognition must be accorded for contributions from the National Dairy Council, the American Dietetic Association, their cooperating state societies, and especially Dr. Jean Robbins, Jane Franklin, and Natalie Dickstein, and from our own Department of Nutrition, especially Gloria Elfert and Millicent Kelly who made valuable contributions to our program. An expression of gratitude to Dr. Ghislaine Godenne, Lee Schatz, and Shirley Tansy, of the Hopkins Homewood Campus division of our program.

Thanks for the outstanding assistance of: the International Flight Attendants Association; its thousands of members; President Peter Tronke of Germany; Past President Advisor Lyne Pike of Australia; and the twenty-seven major airlines here and abroad which have contributed much to the valuable research in our work. My sincere appreciation to Pan American World Airways; its past president, Dan Colussy; Felicia Fairchild and Kathy Williams; to Andrew and Cathy Alexa, of the National Association of Flight Attendants.

I am also indebted to my editor, Nancy Crawford, for her unwavering belief in the importance of this work; to Joan Heilman, my co-author, for the shape, sparkle and clarity her collaboration brought to this book, and to Eleanor Rawson, my publisher, whose encouragement and perceptive analysis have been inspirational.

Preface

Each year the public is deluged with a flood of new diet books, weight-loss plans and get-thin-quick schemes. They find a ready market, catering to an almost universal desire to possess the perfect figure and attain perfect health. Advertisements universally feature successful people who appear svelte and healthy and beautiful.

Amid this profusion of schemes are many that are sound, safe and effective, as well as many that are unsound, dangerous and ineffective. Many plans prescribe one diet plan for all who wish to lose weight, thereby failing to consider individual food tolerances and preferences.

In the midst of this bewildering mass of information Dr. Simonson has brought us a plan geared to the needs of the individual. She has drawn from her fourteen-year experience with the Health, Weight and Stress Program at Johns Hopkins to produce this book. It contains a wealth of sound information on the causes of overweight, its classifications and methods for combating it, emphasizing that in many cases diet alone may not be the whole answer.

Influenced by the teachings of recognized experts in nutrition, medicine and the behavioral sciences, the contents are based on replicated research results and clinical experience with patients. These are programs and techniques that have worked.

Dr. Simonson's program offers advice on both many new and many known aspects of the problem of weight management. Although written for the individual, this book also can be of value to the professional therapist or to anyone interested in a safe and sensible approach to weight control.

Throughout rings a universal truth concerning weight control: Calories in minus calories out equal calories stored or lost. The difficulties inherent in applying this axiom were recognized in the advice of Socrates in 399 B.C.: "Beware of those foods that tempt you to eat when you are not hungry and those liquors that tempt you to drink when you are not thirsty."

Agatha A. Rider, Sc.M.
Assistant Professor
Department of Biochemistry
School of Hygiene and Public Health
The Johns Hopkins University
Baltimore, Maryland

The Complete
University Medical Diet

Before You Begin This Book . . .

Our renowned Health, Weight and Stress Program developed at Johns Hopkins began as a self-help group in 1969, when fifteen overweight employees and faculty members of the Johns Hopkins University School of Hygiene decided they needed help losing weight. I was among them. After trying several lecturers associated with commercial weight-loss groups and discovering that none of them gave us what we needed, we decided to meet on our own. The first thing we did was to elicit advice, assistance and information from the Departments of Medicine, Psychology and Nutrition at Johns Hopkins.

Our strategy worked. We all lost weight, and we kept it off, too, because we treated ourselves as individuals and more than simply eating machines. I, like many others in the group, started out weighing more than 300 pounds and slimmed down to less than half my former size.

Before long some of the Medical Institutions' physicians requested us to include some of their patients in our group, and the Department of Nutrition sent us others who, the dietitians believed, needed more support in their efforts to lose weight than simple nutritional advice.

We recruited physicians, counselors, psychologists, dietitians and other professionals to develop guidelines. Within a year our weight program had become an officially sanctioned extramural group within the university's famous School of Hygiene and Public Health. I became the director.

In 1976, this clinic, conducted by me and now called the Johns Hopkins Health, Weight and Stress Program moved its administrative operations to the Department of Psychiatry where it became part of the health services offered by the department of which I am a faculty member.

HOW THE PROGRAM WORKS

Today 200 to 300 men and women, adolescents and children come to our classes each month, some of them traveling hundreds of miles to attend. From the many classes scheduled they choose the one that meets at a time convenient for them. We even have a "night owl class" that starts at 11:00 P.M. for late-shift workers. Our only prerequisite for entrance into the program is that everyone who joins must be referred by a doctor and have had a physical examination within the last month.

During a two-week orientation period a battery of psychological tests and a consultation with staff therapists help pinpoint emotional problems that directly influence eating habits and perhaps signal the need for counseling. Detailed questionnaires tell us precisely how the patient lives and eats, the family background, previous weight-loss efforts, environmental influences, etc. If necessary, home visits and family interviews are scheduled.

Each person is asked to keep a Food Diary, a record of what is eaten and when, and to answer a food questionnaire designed to review eating habits and reveal possible nutritional imbalances. We then develop a total person profile for each patient, examining the physical, psychological, environmental and nutritional factors that influence his or her weight.

Then, when we know as much as possible about each overweight patient, the university and hospital nutritionists prescribe a diet, individually tailored to each person's specific needs and food preferences.

Our classes are designed to encourage the maximum involvement and self-awareness of each participant. Every class is preceded by a group therapy session led by trained counselors for those who wish to attend. This session provides a powerful tool for getting at the underlying reasons for overeating. For many, perhaps most, of the attendants this is the only place they have ever dared examine their innermost problems as they relate to their weight.

Weekly meetings consist of private weigh-ins, group demonstrations and a series of lectures—by guest speakers as well as our staff, which is professionally trained and accredited—on relevant topics: physiology, nutrition, environmental and social factors, pathogenesis of obesity, psychological aspects of behavior, etc. New techniques are researched, and tests and questionnaires periodically update insights and information.

The result of this extremely thorough multidisciplinary approach to weight loss? Not only do a high percentage of our patients successfully lose weight and learn to keep it off, but they develop an increased awareness of food, better nutritional habits and a healthier, better balanced eating plan than they ever thought possible.

A recent survey of health agencies and health journals showed that our program at this prestigious university and medical center investigated and dealt with more areas of each individual's problem with weight *than any other clinic surveyed.* And it cost approximately 10 percent of the fee charged at any of the commercial diet centers. Many of our patients, because they are economically disadvantaged, pay nothing.

SIDELINES

Our Health, Weight and Stress Program helps not only the hundreds of people who come to the classes every week at Johns Hopkins but, through auxiliary programs, many thousands of others as well. We act as consultants to eleven major industrial firms in five states and to the International Flight Attendants Association, the members of which are drawn from twenty-seven domestic, shuttle and corporate airlines, among them Pan American, United, Eastern, American, TWA, U.S. Air as well as from almost every foreign airline in the world.

And more: We have developed special weight-control plans for many groups, including all branches of the U.S. armed forces and police and fire departments throughout the state of Maryland. Our program has been used as a model for other clinics all over the globe.

Special two-week internships offer training for medical students, nurses, dietitians, psychologists and counselors.

Perhaps most impressive of all, we pioneered the concept of a continuing-education course for professionals in the study of obesity, its causes and treatment. Those attending the one-week course—among them, doctors, nutritionists, psychologists, and allied health professionals—receive accreditation from the American Medical Association, their own universities, and from the Johns Hopkins University.

Other accreditation comes from such professional organizations as the American Dietetic Association, the American Nurses' Association, the American Psychological Association, the Association of Physicians in Family Practice as well as all branches of the United States armed forces, health centers and state health departments and government agencies.

Our yearly professional continuing-education course is held at the Johns Hopkins Medical Institutions in Baltimore every spring with a limited attendance of 160 participants. Guest speakers and instructors are chosen from among the leading authorities on obesity in the world.

It is our sincere hope that the techniques and unique approach to weight loss we employ with such success at Johns Hopkins will prove equally valuable to you in your efforts to lose weight permanently.

Maria Simonson, Ph.D., Sc.D.,Director,
Health, Weight and Stress Program,
the Johns Hopkins Medical Institutions,
Baltimore, Maryland

1. The Famous Weight-Loss Program at Johns Hopkins

Name a diet, I have been on it. And I lost weight, too, but it never lasted very long. Before I knew it, I was just as heavy as I was before I started. It became so discouraging that finally I decided to forget it. It was only after my doctor insisted that I had to lose some weight or face dire consequences that I came to the program here at Johns Hopkins. I now feel in control of myself and my body, and I am losing weight steadily. It's amazing what a difference it makes to confront yourself.

—Thirty-four-year-old schoolteacher

If you have had enough of the place-name diets, the diarrhea diets, the single-food or special-combination diets, the high-protein, the low-carbohydrate, the all-fiber diets, the fasts, the one-week-on, one-week-off diets and are now ready to take the *proven* route to significant weight loss, we offer the program developed at one of the most prestigious universities and medical centers in the United States.

This weight-control plan, originated and developed by our Health, Weight and Stress program, is a total and complete weight-control plan that has been remarkably successful for nearly 40,000 people. It doesn't make extravagant and unwarranted promises. It simply assures success—a loss of a pound or two or more (the more you have to lose, the faster you can lose it) every single week as long as you stay with it. It works whether you have 10 pounds or 250 pounds to lose. It guarantees you will be eating all the essential nutrients your body requires for good health and high energy, and it gives you a far better chance of keeping the pounds off than any of the highly publicized methods, including the most famous and commercially successful.

Our now-famous program has helped thousands of people who

have never before managed—despite their best efforts—to become thinner or permanently thin. Our success rate (based on maintenance of weight loss and other strict criteria) is superior to the claims of many other groups, commercial or private.

Medically documented, our program is a synthesis of the best, safest, most legitimate, most effective techniques of weight loss known today. The opposite of a gimmick fad diet, the antithesis of a crash program, it is the result of fifteen years of solid research and vast experience. And that's the secret of its phenomenal success here in Baltimore and the reason it has become world-renowned. Physicians, nutritionists, biochemists, dietitians and other health professionals from all over the globe come to our continuing-education courses and our classes to learn what really is valid in a field rampant with quackery and unproven claims.

The bizarre diets have had their day. Now it is time for the grown-up approach to weight loss. It is time to be sensible—and to achieve lasting success. Anyone can take weight off, but few can *keep* it off. If you are reading this book, you know how true that is.

The facts are:

There is no magic cure for fat.

There are no shortcuts to thinness.

There is only one way to lose weight: Eat less and exercise more! The problem is how to do that long enough, without feeling inordinately deprived and restrained, to get thinner and stay that way.

"THE DIET THAT SUCCEEDS WHEN ALL OTHERS FAIL"

This was the title of an article about the program at the Johns Hopkins University in *Self* magazine more than a year ago, stating that it was one of the most successful weight-control programs in the country. Though we weren't looking for publicity, we got it. The article prompted one of the highest readers' responses the magazine had ever received: more than 28,000 letters and hundreds of telephone calls from both professional and consumer readers asking for our techniques and special information. Inundated, we requested no more—we couldn't handle it.

Instead, we have decided to share what we do for our patients who come to the program in Baltimore, as well as the employees of twenty-seven international airlines and eleven major industrial firms and dozens of other groups and clinics throughout the country for which we set up and supervise weight-control programs.

Hence, this book.

We have been living through an era of obsession with thinness and the most outrageous, outlandish diets, dangerous diet pills and potions, ineffective or hazardous machines and gadgets, all of which promise to make us thin effortlessly and fast. Americans spend more than $80 million a year searching for painless solutions to a lifelong problem. At the Health, Weight and Stress Program at Johns Hopkins we have collected more than 29,000 methods of losing weight and have found fewer than 6 percent of them to be effective or even safe. Some we wouldn't give to a cigar-store Indian because the wood would deteriorate! Most Americans will do anything to escape being fat.

At any one time about 70 million Americans say they want to lose weight and 9.5 million are in some kind of weight program. Sixty-seven percent of the entire population reports going on one or more diets every year. Nevertheless, the average American weighs more today than ever before. And 9 out of every 10 losers are right back where they started from, and then some, within eight months.

THE SECRET INGREDIENTS
OF THE UNIVERSITY MEDICAL DIET

The University Medical Diet uses self-knowledge as the key to the fight against fat. **The secret is honest self-evaluation, an understanding of who you are and how you function.** You must become closely acquainted with yourself to be a successful loser; that means keeping the lost weight off. If you want to be thin, you must investigate your biology, heritage, life-style, emotions, psychological connections with food and then use this information to overpower your tendency to gain weight.

That's why this program is not just "a diet." And the focus is not on food, menus, recipes. It is a complete and total multidisciplinary program employing hundreds of techniques to help you lose weight, all based on your personal discoveries.

The Demographics of Dieting

Did you know that:

• If you live on the West or East Coast of the United States, you are especially likely to be on a diet or planning one. But as a group, people who live on the two coasts are thinner than those in the mid-Atlantic or midwestern states.

• If you are a woman dieter, you are probably between the ages of eighteen and forty-nine. If you are a man, your age is most likely about forty.

• The people with the highest interest in losing weight have family incomes in the middle or upper brackets.

• A study by Dr. Albert Stunkard of the University of Pennsylvania rates Protestants as the thinnest religious group in the American population. Episcopalians lead the pack, followed by Presbyterians, Methodists and Baptists. Catholics are somewhat plumper than Protestants, while, as a group, the Jews are the heaviest of all.

• First-generation Americans are five times more likely to be heavy than people whose families have been in the United States for several generations.

• The thinnest ethnic groups in the United States come from families originating in England; the weightiest from Poland and Russia.

Our premise is: If you don't understand yourself and what makes you overeat—and it isn't your mother-in-law, your boss or your spouse!—then you aren't dealing with the real issue. You may lose weight, but the "symptom" of fat will return. Your food habits are unique. They are characteristic of you alone, a sum total of your individual experience. You cannot separate your overweight body from the person within it.

The fact is, you will be on one diet and possibly as many as three diets a year, every year, for the rest of your life—if you don't finally become realistic.

QUICK WEIGHT LOSS IS A FRAUD

The University Medical Diet promises a *gradual* and *steady weight loss.* Quick weight loss, though it sounds painless and easy and perhaps even fun, not only is unhealthy and potentially dangerous but doesn't work! The weight you lose on that kind of diet—essentially water, not fat—inevitably comes back, usually just about as fast as it came off.

The reason we stress gradually losing in our program is critical: A gradual weight loss gives you time to know yourself, so you can make changes and adjustments in the way you relate to food. If you try to lose weight in too much of a hurry, you invest too little of yourself to break the bad habits that made you overweight in the first place. And just as important, rapid weight loss does not allow sufficient time to absorb the reality of the influence of biology on your weight. Not only does your body attempt to stay at its accustomed weight, but it is physiologically more difficult for some people to lose weight than it is for others. To develop a realistic long-term plan that will continue to work for you, it's essential to discover and understand your own personal physical obstacles to weight loss.

And there's a bonus: Gradually losing weight helps prevent the tissue damage that advances the signs of aging. **If you follow our guidelines, you will look younger longer.**

WHAT YOU WILL LEARN

In this book, you will learn the answers to questions like these:

· Was your body designed by nature to be overweight?
· How can you overpower your own biological programming?
· Why do you gain weight on the very same calories that make other people lose?
· What kind of overeater are you: a Night Eater, a Binge Eater, a Mid-life Metabolic Gainer, a Gastronomic Overeater or one of many other scientifically researched categories?
· Why do rainy days and red tablecloths tend to make you eat more?
· How do you use food to solve your problems and relieve your tensions?

· Are bananas more fattening than oranges?

· Is whole-wheat bread better than white bread when you are on a weight-loss program?

· Are you an overweight "owl" who skips breakfast, makes up for it in extracurricular snacking in the late afternoon and at night and specializes in high-calorie binges? Or are you an overweight "lark," who leads a more structured life and whose prime time for overeating is in midmorning?

· Do you know you are likely to stop losing weight temporarily around the seventh or eighth week into a diet?

· When is Quitter's Week, the time most people become diet dropouts?

· What are the nineteen best ways to confront an oncoming eating attack and the twenty ways to boggle your mind so you'll lose more efficiently?

· What kind of exercise speeds up metabolism and therefore weight loss?

· What is the best time of day to eat most of your calories?

· Why does your "natural" weight tend to hover around a certain number on the scale?

· How can you get off to a flying start on a diet?

· Why are men more successful than women when it comes to losing weight?

The answers to all these questions are here—and much more. You will find information you never before have read in any book about weight control.

And you will discover who you are as an eater.

THE FOOD PLAN

This book will, of course, include the famous University Medical Diet food plan, which is designed to be individualized according to your own food preferences and eating patterns. You may arrange the calories so you can lose as quickly or as gradually as you like. The diet is based on food trade-offs, nutritional equivalents that allow you to plan your own menus *around the foods you like* without overstepping your calorie boundaries.

It is also based on increased physical activity, especially for those who are biologically programmed to be overweight.

More Weighty Facts

• The average American dieter goes on 2.3 diets a year, lasting sixty to ninety days. Women, considered separately, average 3 diets a year.

• Large numbers of Americans, especially adolescent girls and grown women, who are chronically on low-calorie diets, eat far less than the recommended daily allowances of many essential nutrients, endangering their current and future health. Some of the deficiences found in a nationwide food consumption survey include vitamins A, C and B complex, calcium, iron, magnesium, potassium and phosphorus.

• Studies at our clinic at Johns Hopkins show that the middle-income woman is the hardest of all to help lose weight. Low-income women are more likely to learn helpful nutritional information and use it to change their cooking and eating habits. On the other hand, low-income groups are the fattest. Twenty-five percent of low-income white women and 35 percent of low-income black women are obese.

• Among men, the blue-collar, low-income individual often strenuously resists losing weight, even when he is told his life depends on it. That's because he often equates size with power and unconsciously fears that losing weight will reduce his impact on the world around him.

• Habitual television watchers consume, on average, about one-third more calories a day than people who spend more time on the go. They also exercise the least. A survey of health habits made by the Massachusetts Department of Public Health found that people who watch more than five hours of TV a day are markedly less likely to exercise than others.

• It has been found that 80 percent of the children born to two obese parents, and 41 percent of those born to one obese parent, become overweight themselves. Only 9 percent of the offspring of two thin parents grow up with a weight problem.

The program is designed for high energy and weight loss, a speed-up of your metabolism and a quicker use of calories so they convert into energy rather than fat tissue.

But while the diet is essential, it is not the most important part of our program or this book because, as you surely know by now, *every* diet works. If it provides fewer calories than you have been consuming, you will lose weight, whether it's cream cheese and jelly sandwiches or celery sticks. You can lose even more by exercising. Only calories, consumed and burned, make a difference. Nothing else.

In this book you will learn to manipulate those calories, with the best chance you have ever had to be permanently thin.

2. The Total Person Approach

Whenever, whatever, however you eat, you bring along all your associations, past history, habits, emotions and attitudes. And you bring along your body, which may be doing its best to outwit your efforts to get thin. You carry your nutritional knowledge, your health, your stresses.

At the weight clinic we conduct at Johns Hopkins, we examine the total person, the complete package—you, with all your physiological and psychological baggage. Through questionnaires, tests and interviews, we evaluate and encourage your ability to lose weight. Through counseling, we offer insight. Through lectures, we provide straightforward information and advice. Periodic appointments with the dietitians help you plan your diet. Through this book you can help yourself gain the same benefits.

Only when you understand what you have to work with can you begin to help yourself lose weight permanently. Only when you start to know your *inner* self can you start to control your *outer* self.

So let's begin. Take this Demographic Profile Questionnaire, adapted from the award-winning test given at our clinic. Your answers will give you a true reflection of yourself and your eating personality. It will point out your strengths and weaknesses, the influences on your behavior and your own attitudes.

Think carefully before answering each question. Be honest. If you want to keep your responses confidential, photocopy the questionnaire so that only you will see them. Your evaluations will help you pinpoint your problem areas and make you aware of how you handle—or mishandle—the food in your life.

DEMOGRAPHIC PROFILE QUESTIONNAIRE

You and Your Family

Name _____ Age _____ Sex _____ Height
_____ Weight _____ Body build _____ Ethnic and religious
background _____ Marital status _____
Number of children _____ Do you live alone? _____ With family?
_____ Others? _____ In a house? _____ Apartment? _____
Hotel? _____ Other? _____
How much did you weigh at the following ages?
Birth _____ Age 10 _____ 15 _____ 25 _____ Now _____
Your maximum weight _____ Age _____
Your minimum weight _____ Age _____
How old were you when you first had a "weight problem"? _____
What is your current state of health? _____ What physi-
cal conditions do you have that affect the foods you eat? _____
_____
Describe the following members of your family as thin, average, heavy,
very heavy: Yourself _____ Spouse _____ Mother _____ Father
_____ Sisters _____ Brothers _____ Children _____
Is there someone in your household who likes to cook?
Who? _____

Life-style

How do you spend your time (i.e., working; caring for family; cooking;
sedentary activities, such as studying, reading, watching TV; physical
activities; traveling)? _____
_____
If you work, what is your job? _____
Do you frequently eat away from home? _____ How often?

_____ Why? _____ Do you

smoke? _____ How much? _____ Do you have prob-

lems sleeping? _____ How many hours do you usually sleep?

_____ When? _____ Do you do any kind of regular exer-

cise? _____ Irregular? _____

Are you less physically active today than you once were? _____ What

are your interests and hobbies? _____

_____

Do you often have long stretches of time when you have nothing to do?

_____

Weight Expectations

Why do you want to lose weight? _____

_____

What do you think are your reasons for your overweight? _____

_____

How much do you want to lose? _____

Have you ever planned your own diet? _____

How many times have you tried to lose weight before? _____

How? _____

Were you successful or did you regain? _____

Did you feel you were expected to lose weight too rapidly? _____

Did you feel you were expected to lose more weight than you could?

_____

When you were dieting, did you feel as if you were under increased

pressure? Did you feel deprived, restricted, anxious, hostile, depressed,

insecure? _____

Nutrition and Eating Behavior

Do you feel you have a good appetite? _____

What time of day are you most hungry? _____

Are you hungry before meals? _____

What times do you usually eat your meals? Breakfast _____ Lunch _____ Dinner _____

Do you eat fruit every day? _____ How much? _____

Do you eat vegetables every day? _____ How much? _____

Do you eat cereals and whole grains? _____ How much? _____

Do you drink milk or eat milk products? _____ How much? _____

How many cups of coffee and/or tea do you drink in a day? _____

Do you add milk or sugar? _____

How many soft drinks do you have in a day? _____ Regular _____ Low-calorie _____

Do you drink alcoholic beverages? How much? _____ How often? _____

What is your total fluid intake per day? 1 quart? _____ Less? _____ 2 quarts? _____ 1 gallon or more? _____

Do you think you understand the basic principles of nutrition? _____

Do you think you	Yes	No	Sometimes
1. Overeat?	—	—	_____
2. Get too little exercise?	—	—	_____
3. Understand nutrition but don't apply it?	—	—	_____
4. Nibble rather than eat three meals a day?	—	—	_____
5. Eat the wrong foods?	—	—	_____
6. Other?	—	—	_____

Do you ever estimate your daily caloric intake? _____

Can you do it correctly? _____ Number of calories? _____

Do you have strong food preferences?

Likes? _____

Dislikes? _____

Do you have specific associations with certain foods? What are they?

How many *meals* per day do you normally eat? _____

How often do you snack? _____ What do you eat for snacks? _____

_____

Do you choose foods because of:

1. Habit? _____
2. Environmental conditions (work, family, etc.)? _____
3. Stress? _____
4. Taste, sight, craving? _____
5. Ethnic or cultural conditioning? _____
6. Hunger? _____
7. Social pressures? _____
8. Time pressures? _____
9. Travel? _____
10. Other? _____

WHAT YOUR ANSWERS TELL YOU

What have you learned from your answers? How would you describe the kind of eater you are? Does any of the information in your responses surprise you?

For example, in the section "You and Your Family," you may have learned that you are following your family's tradition of overeating and overweight or that your problem with pounds began earlier in your life than you realized. The way you live— alone, with a family, in a home, a hotel—obviously influences your eating, though you may not have considered its impact before. When you eat most of your meals at home, you will have better control over your calories, but at the same time more temptations on your shelves. When you live with your family, you must think of their needs as well as your own, and their eating habits may rub off on you.

"Life-style": The amount of physical activity that's required as you go about your daily routine, and how much you add in purposeful exercise, have a profound effect on your weight. So be as active as you can; cultivate your interests and hobbies. People who are bored tend to eat more. If your chief interest is watching television with a bowl of pretzels by your side, you are going to be fatter than if you spend much of your spare time crocheting afghans, riding a horse or building furniture.

"Weight Expectations": To lose weight successfully, your motivation must be high, it must persist long enough for you to get thin and stay that way and your goals must be realistic. If none of these factors check out, you are going to abandon your weight-loss efforts before you give yourself a real chance.

"Nutrition and Eating Behavior": Your answers to the questions in this section will tell you whether you eat healthily and rationally, whether you know the facts about nutrition and apply them. You will get a clue, too, to the major reasons why you eat *what* you eat *when* you eat it. If you don't eat enough of the essential body-building foods, and fill up on concentrated calories instead, you will not only gain weight but risk your health as well. See Chapters 9 and 10 for helpful information about food and how you eat it.

In the next chapter you will discover even more about your eating personality and why you are overweight. The descriptions of the five basic eating personalities and thirteen psychological types of overeaters will help you find out more exactly who you are as an eater.

3. Profiles in Overweight: Which Type Are You?

Eating makes me feel better. It's like a friend. Sure, I know I'll feel awful about it later on, but at that moment when I'm feeling down or angry about something, it seems to be the only thing that helps. The last time I really went hog-wild was on a Saturday night. All my friends had dates, even my parents had gone out to dinner and there I was all alone, feeling unwanted and unloved. I ate four hot dogs and two grilled cheese sandwiches, and then, half an hour later, I ate almost a whole bag of cookies and drank three glasses of milk. That was on top of a big dinner.

—Nineteen-year-old student

Dr. Frank Bigsby, former senior faculty member of the Tulane University School of Medicine and an authority on the clinical management of obesity, says, "You can't discuss the treatment of overweight in general terms. That's like talking about the treatment of all diseases under the title 'Treatment of Sickness.' "

We all are different, and the reasons we are overweight are unique to each one of us. However, from our surveys over the last fifteen years at the clinic at Johns Hopkins University of thousands of overweight people of all ages, occupations, and backgrounds, we have discovered certain patterns among them. **We have identified these patterns and grouped them—with the help of Dr. Bigsby—into four basic profiles and thirteen psychological types of overeaters. These categories will help you pinpoint the kind of overeater you are—**a crucial point for weight loss because you cannot fight your weight problem realistically if you don't know what it is.

You will find that one profile or type will describe you best— this is your primary group—but you will overlap into others. For example, you may have some of the characteristics of the Compulsive Eater as well as the Night Eater and have a constitutionally large body build as well. Or you may be a Mid-life Gainer who began as a Sedentary Overeater. Once you know where you fit, you will be better able to deal with your unique situation.

The categories include those that are essentially physiological: constitutional or body type, hormonal and organic, as well as the kinds of overweight typical in childhood or mid-life. **But by far the greatest number of people who weigh too much are the Psychological Overeaters, who use food to solve their emotional problems. In fact, our surveys have shown that this category comprises 85 percent of the entire overweight population in America,** though it is usually superimposed on a body build predisposed to weight gain. According to our studies at the university, there are thirteen major psychological types of overeaters. Read the descriptions based on our findings to help you determine your dominant type.

First, however, you must know how your body build affects your weight. The basic profiles follow.

1. BODY TYPE OR CONSTITUTIONAL OVERWEIGHT

If you are constitutionally overweight, you have inherited a frame that is large and/or a body that encourages the storage of fat in your supersupply of expandable fat cells.

A generally accepted method of characterizing genetically determined body shapes was originated back in 1940 by Dr. William H. Sheldon, a physician and psychologist who meticulously studied the shapes of more than 45,000 people. Called somatotypes, his categories describe three basic body builds: ectomorph, mesomorph and endomorph. Few of us are pure examples of one type, but we all tend to be more one than another.

· The *ectomorph*—whom we'll pass by quickly because you are not one if you are reading this book—has a thin, linear body, with delicate, attenuated bones, slim muscles, long, narrow feet and hands and the largest skin surface area in proportion to body mass of the three body types. The person with this body can pile on the calories and never gain weight. Some ectomorphs are tremendous eaters yet never show it. They may, in fact, have great difficulty maintaining a healthy and attractive body weight and may be just as miserable about it as the rest of us are about our propensity to weigh too much.

Dr. Sheldon found ectomorphs are inclined to be restrained and inhibited, cerebral, intense, youthful and quick.

· The classic *mesomorph* has a firm, sturdy or muscular body that tends to be rectangular in shape, with heavy bones, a large chest, prominent bone joints, broad hands and well-developed shoulder and leg muscles.

This kind of person, though sometimes hippy, is usually broader at the top than the bottom, tends to stand up straight and frequently is not as overweight as he or she may seem. In fact, he or she may not have much surplus fat at all on those big bones; mesomorphs are seldom obese. Many, though they think they are overweight, actually have only a healthy percentage of fat content and should not attempt to diet themselves down to an unrealistic size, which they probably cannot achieve or can accomplish only with constant deprivation and the danger of consuming fewer calories than necessary for a high level of energy and health.

Sheldon characterized mesomorphs as basically vigorous, assertive and youthful with a love of exercise and adventure.

Most mesomorphs come from families originating in the countries of northern Europe, such as Russia, Poland, Scandinavia, and as children they were always larger than their playmates.

They usually eat regular balanced meals that include a fair amount of starches and other carbohydrates. Their eating centers around social activities or times of relaxation at home in the evening. They eat in a hurried, businesslike fashion, though they thoroughly enjoy their food. As tests at our clinic have shown, they may not view themselves as large at all.

· Predominantly *endomorphic* people are soft and round and tend to get fat very easily. They often have relatively small facial features, broad upper arms and prominent abdomens. And they float high in the water! That's because they store a higher percentage of fat in their bodies than the other two basic body types.

Endomorphs usually love comfort, people, affection—and *food.* According to Sheldon, they tend to be relaxed and sociable. They're the ones who usually bring the cakes, bake the cookies, cook up a feast when company's coming. For them, offering food may be an expression of love.

Most people who become very much overweight are endomorphs.

2. ORGANIC AND HORMONAL OVERWEIGHT

A second variety of physiological overweight is the kind that results from a physical abnormality, and it is extremely rare. Though it's long been an American tradition to blame our glands for our fat, fewer than 6 percent of the entire obese population belong in this category. It's an excuse that's going out of style as we gather more evidence that it simply isn't so very often.

Among the extremely unusual causes of organic obesity are brain injuries or lesions and pituitary tumors. Occasionally, too, a serious malfunction of the endocrine glands contributes to the overweight by influencing the body's caloric balance, and true hypoglycemia has been the cause of extreme weight gains in some instances.

Some glandular disorders produce the formation of fat pads in characteristic areas of the body because they affect the distribution of fat. In Cushing's disease, for example, the face becomes moon-shaped, and fat pads develop in the thighs, the hips and the back of the neck. People with lipodystrophy may have very thin upper bodies but very large hips and legs. Fröhlich's disease causes an unequal distribution of fat, accumulating mainly in the thighs and around the waistline.

The gland that has always been blamed the most for excess fat is the thyroid. This gland does play a vital part in maintaining stable body weight, though only a small number of obese people can claim the distinction of being heavy because of it. If it is your problem, your doctor will probably spot it immediately because the symptoms of a real deficiency are characteristic: a large accumulation of weight in the upper body, puffy face and eyelids and a dry, coarse, pale skin.

On the other hand—we'll discuss this in detail shortly—glandular disturbances may be a *consequence* of persistent serious overweight, making it all the harder to lose. Usually these disturbances eventually will return to normal after a sizable weight loss, but sometimes they always remain slightly out of kilter.

3. MID-LIFE METABOLIC OVERWEIGHT

The people who acquire most of their extra poundage when they reach middle age fit into their own special listing because the cause is both physiological and psychological. In mid-life not only do you usually lead a more sedentary life and focus more on food and the enjoyment of eating than you did when you were young, but you may have physical problems that influence your food selection.

Besides, you now require fewer calories to maintain your body at a constant weight. The older you are, the lower your basal metabolism rate is likely to be. That means your body doesn't need as much fuel to keep it going, and the excess calories are stored as fat. The body's percentage of fat tissue in relation to lean muscle tissue increases as the years go by. Fat tissue uses fewer calories than muscle tissue simply to exist, and fewer as well are burned off. It is only logical that if you continue to eat as you always have, you will put on weight, especially if you don't get much exercise.

So you are *now* an overeater, even though you have not changed your habits, because you consume more than your body needs.

Do Added Years
Mean Added Pounds?

• Your basal metabolism slows down about 3 percent from age twenty-two to thirty-five; then, with each passing decade, it decreases at an escalating rate. If you are far overweight, you lose energy three to eight years earlier than normal. Since you also acquire a higher percentage of accumulated fat tissue in relation to lean body mass as you get older, you'll need fewer and fewer calories to stay static.

• The average adult who is fifteen pounds overweight by middle age got that way by adding one to five pounds a year between the ages of twenty-eight and forty-two.

• At forty-five, you should weigh what you did at twenty-six if you weren't overweight.

This is especially true for women whose falling estrogen production affects their weight and their figures. As estrogen diminishes, women tend to gain and, at the same time, become less curvy and more straight up and down, losing fat in the hips, thighs and breasts and gaining it in the back, rib cage and waistline.

Middle-aged men tend to gain most in their midsections.

While men in their younger years can lose weight twice as fast as women (see next chapter), they begin losing some of their advantage over the opposite sex when they reach middle age because of their declining percentage of muscle and increasing ratio of fat tissue.

To make matters worse for both men and women, the muscles and tissue membranes as well as the skin lose some of their elasticity and so do not hold the fat tissue as tightly as they once did.

Mid-life weight gain is seldom excessive unless you have previously been obese, in which case you may balloon once more. Our studies show that, as a mid-life gainer, your motivation to stay with a diet until you lose sufficient weight is usually excellent.

4. JUVENILE OVERWEIGHT

There are two distinct kinds of juvenile or adolescent overweight, and we call them puberal and developmental.

Puberally overweight youngsters are characterized by a sudden and pronounced spurt of growth, maturation and size as they approach puberty, and they usually remain heavy for two or three years. Their eating pattern tends to be regular and includes real meals, but it is highlighted by typical teen-age eating behavior, with an emphasis on between-meal snacks of starches and sweets. Teen-agers don't overeat primarily because of emotional tension or anxiety but out of habit and a desire to be like their peers.

Fortunately most puberally obese youngsters are blessed with understanding parents and a fair amount of emotional stability, and once they develop the motivation to eat more sensibly, most of them can lose weight quite easily. But without the proper nutritional and psychological support, they may go on to have more serious difficulties with weight.

Developmentally obese youngsters, however, have more profound problems, both emotional and physical. They are compulsive eaters, snacking and nibbling day and night, rarely eating regular meals, never seeming to be filled up and satisfied, never able to deny themselves the panacea of food for their anxieties, frustrations and low self-esteem.

Usually overweight for as long as they can remember and filled with feelings of inadequacy and unworthiness, developmentally overweight youngsters have an inability to tolerate frustration or a delay in gratification. Their body image is the lowest. They feel something outside themselves forces them to eat, and they have no control over it, though they hate to be fat.

Their home life is usually a morass of misunderstanding, nagging, criticism, sometimes combined with overprotection, emanating from parents (or more often a single parent) with their own emotional problems. A surprising number of their mothers themselves are on diets or, once fat, have become fanatic about their own and their children's needs to be thin, though their attitudes produce the opposite effect.

Developmentally overweight youngsters tend to withdraw from social activities because they feel rejected and undesirable, and at the same time they often become angry, aggressive and rebellious, especially against their parents or other adults who try to help them.

While the puberally overweight adolescent is usually cooperative and eager to collaborate in a weight-loss program once he or she decides it is necessary, the developmentally overweight youngster, in most cases, requires some psychotherapy to help solve the psychological barriers to a more rational eating pattern.

5. PSYCHOLOGICAL OVERWEIGHT—
THE THIRTEEN MAJOR TYPES:

If you use food as a response to your emotional, social and psychological problems, you belong to the largest category of overeaters. In the surveys we made at Johns Hopkins, we have discovered, as noted, that about 85 percent of all overweight people have grown to their current size because they react to almost everything by stuffing food into their mouths. This is especially true, of course, when they also have bodies that are biologically inclined to put on and retain fat. Food is used by psychological overeaters as comfort, tranquilizer, tension reliever, a release for anger, an "upper" for depression and boredom—in fact, as the temporary cure or distraction for whatever bothers them.

Of course, you don't have to be overweight to use food for these purposes; even thin people rely on it. Occasionally almost everyone turns to food as a problem solver. But those of us who gain considerable weight because of it have not yet learned to keep it under control.

The thirteen major types of psychological overeaters are described below. Chances are very good that you will recognize yourself in one or more of them. Where do you fit? Once you understand how you use food and start to notice the signs of imminent overeating, you can begin the task of changing your eating pattern permanently from one that encourages overweight to one that will make you *thin.* Awareness is half the battle in your fight against fat.

The Night Eaters.

Night Eaters, named by Dr. Albert Stunkard, usually consume very little food, or no more than a normal amount, during the day but cannot stop nibbling after dinner. They may even skip breakfast or lunch, providing themselves with a handy rationalization for overeating at night.

Some start nibbling right after the evening meal. They get up from the table and hunt for something tasty to munch on. Then they are summoned by a chair or a couch that silently murmurs, "Come eat with me and watch TV." They respond, chewing all the way. "After all," they think, "I've hardly eaten a thing all day."

Other after-dinner stuffers don't really get going full tilt until the middle of the evening, and then they like to eat as a family group, relaxed and sociable. They start asking, "What have we got to eat?" or "Is there any more of that good chocolate cake?" The evening snack is often a signal to themselves that all's right with their world. We have found that 55 percent of the Night Eaters in our classes fit into this group. Some prefer taking their food up to bed with them. Armed with a piece of cake, a glass of milk, a cheese sandwich, they munch propped up in the pillows. For these people, their snacks are the equivalent of sleeping pills.

Finally, let's consider the *late late* Night Eaters who come in several varieties. These are the people you see in TV commercials, peering into the refrigerator, a chicken leg in one hand, a milk bottle in the other, while a little dog stands on its hind legs, begging for scraps. In bed they toss and turn, then get up to prowl around the kitchen, looking for a bite to eat.

Though there is the small possibility they may really be hungry or suffering from transitory hypoglycemia (low blood sugar), it is much more likely that they are looking for a psychological fix. These are usually people fraught with tensions, fears and anxieties. They can't get to sleep, or they wake up at odd hours, feeling overwhelmed by their problems. Others don't get into the worrying syndrome but simply wake up out of habit, take a stroll to the kitchen for some nutrition and go back to bed, often remembering little about it the next day. One male member of our group gained eleven pounds in three months on middle-of-the-night forays, which he only vaguely recollected until his wife accosted him with pork chop bones and empty soda bottles.

As a group the Night Eaters do not eat three balanced meals a day. Then they feel they can get away with anything because they have been "virtuous" all day. On diets they tend to choose the most outrageous crash regimens because good nutrition usually means little to them. Many are heavy smokers and big coffee consumers as well, and a surprising number spend much of their time traveling for their jobs.

Night Eaters usually love sugary, sweet foods and sometimes spicy dishes, too. Their stress levels measure from borderline to the highest possible level.

Compulsive Eaters.

These overeaters are always munching, nibbling, chomping, and are rarely without something in their mouths. Frequently Compulsive Eaters are closet eaters, sneaking food when nobody is around to observe them. These people use food as a tool to help construct a barrier against anxieties and fears or to form a substitute for what is missing in their lives. It is often equated with love. As one of our patients said, "My stomach doesn't know the difference between food and love."

Food is sometimes used by Compulsive Eaters as a tool or a weapon, a way to get back at themselves for real or imagined sins or inadequacies.

As a group Compulsive Eaters have no organized eating habits and rarely sit down through an entire meal, often eating sparingly at normal eating times, only to snack on the run at all other times. They never throw food away and finish everything and so have been derisively called "human garbage pails." This type is not overly concerned with the quality of the food. Eating is simply a habit.

Favorite foods include sweets and starches and soft, creamy consistencies, as well as liquids, especially diet sodas, but nothing is refused if that's all that is available.

Outwardly many Compulsive Eaters seem to be quite cheerful, though often their outward cheer masks bleak feelings within. Their compulsion to eat hides considerable tension, perhaps the highest level of all the psychological types of overeaters. Food is like a drug to which they are addicted. Unfortunately Compulsive Eaters have little real insight into their emotional problems and how their eating habits are connected to them. Most join weight groups because of pressure from their doctors or families, though sometimes the reason is a feeling that their lives are out of control.

The Liquid Drinkers.

Closely related to Compulsive Eaters are the Liquid Drinkers, who get most of their calories from fluids rather than from solid food. Some consume many quarts of fluids a day, ranging from water and coffee to milk shakes, sodas and alcohol. Unless they drink calorie-rich liquids, their overweight may be mainly due to water-laden tissues rather than to fat. Diet sodas, for example, contain a high percentage of sodium, which promotes water retention.

Liquid Drinkers like to gulp fluids at any time of day, and a glass or a cup in the hand becomes a fixture. They are often workaholics who work under high tension, rarely relaxing and having fun. When they eat, they may choose sandwiches or pieces of pie, doughnuts or fast foods, washed down with two or three cups of coffee or a few cans of soda. Often under considerable stress, they become so addicted to drinking that they have difficulty restraining themselves.

Liquid Drinkers are frequently very overweight, usually wish to be thinner but have minimal insight into their problems and may lack the motivation to stick with a diet plan. Because they often fill themselves up with nonnourishing fluids like diet sodas and black coffee, they often deprive themselves of essential nutrition as well as fiber.

The Binge Eaters.

Though Binge Eaters can go along eating sensibly for hours, days, even weeks, they get sudden urges to eat. Once they start, they don't stop until half a cake is gone, the bag of doughnuts is finished, the refrigerator is cleaned out, or all three.

These overeaters eat rapidly, and they eat steadily, with little regard for table manners or utensils, and when it's over, they usually feel much more relaxed. The binge has served its purpose—the release of tension. But it usually doesn't take long before the relaxation is replaced by a tremendous amount of guilt and self-contempt, which brings on *more* eating as self-punishment or the imposition of a new Spartan regimen of crash dieting or even fasting.

The sudden, unplanned, uncontrolled binges are almost always precipitated by stress or anxiety, often by a specific upsetting occurrence, though the triggering feelings may be carefully buried under a stack of rationalizations. Hostility, anger and depression are among the most usual sources.

Three times as many women as men are Binge Eaters, averaging three sessions of uncontrolled eating per month. The feasting, which is only briefly enjoyable, usually results in a stomach ache and disturbed sleep. It occurs most often late in the evening, sometimes during the night and almost invariably in private. These people are closet eaters, who usually choose sweets and other carbohydrates for the occasion.

Between binges, these overeaters are just like the rest of us, plain overweight people trying to cut back on their daily rations.

NOTE: The above description applies only to garden-variety Binge Eaters. But there is a growing number of people who carry binge eating to astonishing extremes. These are the bulimics, whose eating behavior is so bizarre that they are taking grave risks with their health and even their lives. Bulimics eat tremendous amounts of food, then force themselves to throw up or swallow large amounts of laxatives in an effort to neutralize the food.

Bulimics, who have a serious and dangerous disorder, are more than 95 percent women, most of them very young. They average ten binges a week. Like anorexics, they are obsessed with being thin and are seldom truly overweight. They should consult a medical specialist before they do themselves irreparable harm.

The Expectant Fathers' Syndrome.

It is well documented that women often start on their careers as overweight individuals when they become pregnant, getting heavier with each succeeding child. This is a time when many women indulge themselves with excessive food because they think the fetus is draining them of strength, looks, sex appeal. Or sometimes they are anxious about the pregnancy or the changes in their life-styles. Though they consider weight gain a temporary phenomenon, their new habits may become lifelong patterns.

A surprising fact we have discovered at the Johns Hopkins clinic is that **many men also first become overweight during their wives' pregnancies.** Feelings of rejection or displacement can set off eating binges. No longer the center of attention, perhaps forced to fend for themselves or even help with household chores, resentful of new restrictions on their freedom or worried about new responsibilities, these men find that food makes them feel better, and often they continue to overeat ever after.

Among our members in the last three years the average weight gain of men in this category was thirty-seven pounds in nine months. Usually eating compulsively, the Expectant Father Gainer is likely to be a rather dependent, perhaps emotionally immature young man who finds incipient fatherhood an emotional threat or burden that makes him feel inadquate, insecure, neglected or rejected.

The Traditional Overeaters.

These people have families that have passed along eating habits that are not designed to maintain slim bodies. So you could say they have inherited their fat, but really what they have inherited is a family tradition of overeating.

In most cases the whole family eats the same way, consuming overly large portions and emphasizing calorie-rich foods. They eat substantial breakfasts, good lunches and extravagant dinners, filling in the spaces between with delectable snacks. The well-filled larder, often the result of ethnic influence, is a symbol of security and family love and a link with the past.

Any occasion, however minor, is an excuse for a feast, and life tends to revolve around social activities which revolve around eating. Almost 15 percent of the overweight population comes from this kind of family background.

If you are a member of a "fat family," you probably don't overeat to calm your nerves or ease your frustrations. You eat the way you have been trained to eat at home. You have simply adopted your family's habits. You are likely to be an excellent cook—or married to one. You probably find it extremely difficult to resist the family specialties or the pressure to preserve the traditional patterns. And you may have run into formidable opposition, perhaps unconscious but powerful, when you have decided to change your eating habits in order to lose weight.

The pattern of overeating that you learned from your family is probably accompanied by a decided bias against physical activity, and you get your most strenuous exercise reaching for the pasta or the apple strudel.

The Lipophobics.

Almost exclusively women, the Lipophobics (a word coined by Dr. Bigsby to describe people with an excessive fear of fat) are actually *afraid* of gaining weight. They consider it a sign of weakness and an invitation to disaster. They are obsessed with their weight and have a highly developed talent for talking about the weight gains of their family and friends. We are including them in the psychological types of eaters not because they are often overweight—in fact, they are usually much too *thin*—but because they *think* they are fat and turn up in weight-loss classes in significant numbers.

Lipophobics don't starve themselves as do anorexics, who often eat so little that their health or even their lives are threatened, but they rigidly adhere to their extremely low-calorie meals, trying to make sure everyone around them does, too. They tend to make life for their families extremely difficult because they demand too much of themselves and others. They are perfectionistic and easily frustrated. Sometimes, as a direct result of their insistence on conformity and weight watching, their children become overeaters. Many obese adolescents and young adults have Lipophobic mothers.

Lipophobics have excellent control of their appetites and are often authorities on calorie counts and nutrition. On the other hand, they frequently do not use their knowledge to their own advantage but turn to crash diets indiscriminately because being thin is much more important to them than being healthy.

Also known as thin-fats, Lipophobics usually were once overweight—probably as teenagers. They are now slim but continue to be haunted by the specter of overwhelming flab.

The few Lipophobic men we have encountered tend to be even more obsessively preoccupied with their weight than the women.

The Gastronomic Overeaters.

The Gastronomics are not so much concerned about the quantity of food they eat as with its quality and method of preparation. They are entranced by the delicate nuances of taste. Most Gastronomic Overeaters love to cook because they enjoy the subtleties of flavor and aroma, and they are delighted to demonstrate their expertise in the kitchen. Entertaining at home is their favorite occupation. They never just fix a meal. Instead, it's a matter of pride to prepare something special, even if it's a simple lamb chop with parsleyed potatoes and spinach stir-fried with garlic.

These gourmet eaters rarely eat huge amounts of food and seldom eat between meals, but faced with a delectable delight, they disregard the calories. Gastronomic Overeaters don't eat because of stress and tension, but simply because good food gives them such pleasure. Eating slowly, savoring each forkful, they consciously relish their sensual responses to food.

Sweets don't necessarily appeal to them. If they drink alcohol, they usually prefer wines and liqueurs, both of which may be high in calories. The men in this group—a high percentage of Gastronomic Overeaters is male—are, in general, intellectuals with middle or high incomes and often single or divorced. Both men and women tend to be professionals and in good health.

Few of them are likely to become excessively overweight unless their constitutional body types cannot withstand the overload of calories. Typically their weight gain creeps up on them until, in their mid-forties or fifties, they discover they've become thick around the middle or heavy around the hips.

The Chronic Dieter.

You always know immediately when you are dealing with a Chronic Dieter because she (only occasionally is it a "he") knows everything about dieting and still can't lose weight successfully. She knows better than you do about all diets, knows exactly why she gained weight (again and again), is an expert in nutrition and psychology and can rattle off the calorie count for almost any food from memory. She specializes in trying to prove to you that whatever you suggest won't work for her. She has already tried it.

The problem is that she is also overweight. She knows the answers but doesn't apply them to herself, except in short bursts. She may manage to lose weight but always reverts to her former shape as a result of blaming the regimen, the doctor, the teacher, even the present presidential administration!

The Chronic Dieter, usually a woman in her late thirties or early forties, has gone from doctor to doctor, weight group to weight group, diet book to diet book, and finds them all deficient. She is rarely obese but is usually quite overweight. Similar to the Lipophobic, she is often temperamentally rigid, quick to criticize and instruct other people. She wants immediate results—in time for the party or the Caribbean cruise. She specializes in fad diets, sometimes three or four a year, and is an excellent source of income for manufacturers of diet pills and reducing gadgets. In fact, she will do almost anything except really come to grips with the realities of her overweight body.

Known in weight-control circles as "crazy eaters," Chronic Dieters alternate their fad diets with periods of overeating, gorging on the foods they really love, never missing meals or an opportunity to snack. When guilt sets in once more, it's on to the latest diet or the newest and best publicized (though unproven) miracle method.

The Nutritional Overeaters.

Nutritional Overeaters become overweight simply because they are ignorant about nutrition and don't know what good healthy foods or meals are. Sometimes they don't care to know, or they ignore the facts because they prefer to indulge themselves with the foods they like. They don't know—or refuse to contemplate—what their erratic diets are doing to their health. They are the ones most likely to fall for unhealthy crash diets and gimmicks, always looking for the wonderful diet that lets them eat everything and still lose a pound a day. They just want to lose weight fast.

The Nutritional Overeaters are full of misconceptions about food, are the chief consumers of appetite pills and "diet" powders and supplements and think that vitamins taken indiscriminately will compensate for any gaps in their intake. Fruits and vegetables are never considered of much importance to them; ordinarily they eat them only occasionally and in small amounts.

Nutritional Overeaters are especially prevalent among students and young working women, many of whom never eat real meals but delude themselves into believing they are cutting down their calorie intake by eating little snacks here and there. Unfortunately the snacks add up to plenty of calories and often to a totally unbalanced diet. Many Nutritional Overeaters assiduously avoid carbohydrates (the healthful varieties of which should make up at least 50 percent of one's diet) and fill up on huge amounts of fats and protein. Others specialize in sweets.

Often these overeaters skip breakfast, substituting coffee and cigarettes, and sometimes skip lunch as well. As a result, they frequently experience symptoms of dietary-induced hypoglycemia (low blood sugar)—fatigue, light-headedness, etc.—in late morning and/or late afternoon and compensate with empty calories.

Another favorite trick of Nutritional Overeaters is to rely on diet drinks, granola and yogurt in their efforts to slim down. But they frequently make up for their sacrifices by consuming large dinners and pigging out on sweets, such as Danishes and doughnuts, that arrive temptingly on the cart each morning during coffee break or on the cookies they bought for the rest of the family.

Many in this group eat erratically and poorly because of hectic schedules or because their school hours or jobs preclude regular eating schedules. Rather than plan healthy meals around their daily timetables, they succumb to the pressure through nutritional ignorance or indifference.

The Environmental Eaters.

Their greatest incentive to overeat is in response to the world around them. We all are influenced and even pressured to eat by other people, advertisements, social events, availability of food, sights and smells, but the Environmental Eaters can't resist.

Social life in our culture revolves around food and drink, and all special occasions require refreshments. Bridge parties mean coffee and cake, weddings a six-course dinner; retirement brings not only a gold watch but a big lunch that includes chicken Kiev and ice cream. Business deals are consummated over the dining table, and food is served even at funerals.

It is impossible to turn the pages of a magazine and avoid advertisements of luscious and irresistible food in full color or to snap on the television set and hear about it while we watch somebody devour it. Environmental Eaters, more than others, are turned on by these cues as well as shop windows, fast-food signs, bakery smells. For them, eating is controlled by external stimuli. If they see food, smell it, hear it, think about it, or it's simply available, they eat it, not because of stress or tension but because it is there. They are easily swayed.

Our surveys have found that as a group Environmental Eaters are not excessively overweight, merely more padded than they wish to be. Their problems with weight usually begin with a moderate gain in their early thirties, and then the weight slowly accumulates—around the waistline for men and on the hips and arms for women.

Environmental Eaters are often active in social, civic and business activities at which food plays an important role and tend to be executives, shift workers, working women. They usually love to entertain because they attach such importance to the role of food in their professional and personal relationships. In general, the environmentally influenced overeater is an impulse eater, but also consumes regular meals with larger than average portions.

The Sedentary Gainers.

Members of this overeating group are physically inactive, which causes their initial weight gain. Then, because they are now overweight, they remain inactive and gain even more. Sedentary Gainers are caught in a vicious circle. Many in this group are ex-athletes who once spent hours a day working their muscles. Now they lead more sedentary lives, perhaps behind desks, but they continue to eat like football players. Others, both men and women, spent their earlier years pursuing active school or social lives, but now the most action they get is lifting a fork to their mouths. And even more never exercised much at all, but as they get older and require fewer calories for basal metabolism, it becomes much more difficult for them to maintain a steady weight without exercise.

Sedentary weight gain is closely related, of course, to occupation. Office or factory workers, shop clerks, dentists, even policemen who spend most of their time in patrol cars don't get sufficient physical activity on the job, while door-to-door salespeople, waitresses, forest rangers, manual laborers may get all they need without making special plans to arrange it.

An additional problem: Having put on a lot of weight, the Sedentary Gainers now find it difficult to move easily, so exercise becomes a tremendous exertion and even more of a turnoff. And if they are very overweight, they frequently feel ashamed and embarrassed to be seen exercising because of the way they think they look. Meantime, they continue to get heavier.

Convalescent Overeaters.

Suddenly and not very surprisingly, people who have always had little trouble staying in shape discover that after an illness, an accident or a surgical operation, they expand like balloons.

Obviously a lack of accustomed physical activity is a major reason for a weight gain when you are lying about or sitting in the house with your leg in a cast. Accompanied by no cut in calories, it adds pounds. To add to the problem, many people use their convalescence as a vacation from reality—"I can't get out; the least I can do is eat what I want." Some enjoy the vacation and indulge themselves happily, while others use food to relieve the boredom, depression or frustrations they feel because of the unaccustomed restrictions on their lives.

Our surveys at the Johns Hopkins Medical Institutions have shown that of the people whose normal life-styles are disrupted during a recuperation, 64 percent overeat. Women gain weight during such trying times, but men, we have found, far outnumber them. And a third of these continue to overeat long after they have completely recovered.

Have you identified your eating personality? This exercise in self-examination is the first step toward your goal of losing excess weight successfully. In the ensuing chapters, you will find out exactly how to deal with your particular characteristics.

4. Why Can't a Woman Be More Like a Man?

I'd never admit to my family or anyone else that I eat so much when I get upset. My husband feels if you know enough to talk about it, you can control it. That's not true. When I get feeling unhappy or overwhelmed or frustrated, it doesn't matter why, I get hungry and eat whatever's around. He says things don't affect him like that, he *stops* eating when he's upset, but we're not the same.

—Forty-two-year-old hospital worker

Why can't a woman be more like a man? More people than Professor Higgins, especially women who can't seem to keep their weight down, have wondered about that. In our clinic we constantly hear statements like "But I eat much less than my husband, and he's thin as a rail" or "We both went on the same diet—he lost, and I didn't." And "He can't understand why I can't just stop eating. He can do it anytime he wants. But even when I do cut back, I don't lose very much."

When it comes to weight, men are by far the superior beings. As a general rule, it is much easier for men to be thin. Fewer of them ever get fat, to begin with. That's mainly because their bodies naturally contain more muscle tissue in relation to fat tissue than women's do. Though they may weigh more, less of their weight is fat. Besides, they can lose weight much more rapidly.

Most girls start gaining fat tissue, very often much to their sorrow, during adolescence because one of the major functions of the female hormone estrogen is to promote the storage of fat in preparation for pregnancy. Men, on the other hand, usually *lose* weight during adolescence (later for men than for women) since one of testosterone's chief purposes is to favor the development of muscles.

Perhaps because they see results more quickly, when men

decide to shed pounds, they are much more likely than women to accomplish their goal—without the emotional turmoil and backing and filling that usually accompany the process among women. Though some men have biochemical flaws that make them put on fat easily, and many have body types that were designed by nature to be rotund, **most men have enormous physiological and psychological advantages over women.**

BATTLING FAT AND THE DOUBLE STANDARD

First of all, the double standard rears its unattractive head. **Fat is, for the most part, a woman's issue. Men are far less affected by being overweight.** Their shapes—unless they become truly extreme—seldom influence their self-esteem or the respect of others. Men are not usually viewed as unattractive, undisciplined or out of control until they reach far larger proportions than women do. Though overweight, men are not considered "fat," but "powerful," "large," "stocky," "portly." When they lose weight, it is usually for health reasons. And for most men, overweight arrives in middle age, so their sense of identity has already been firmly fixed before fat enters their lives.

But women don't get off so easily. They see themselves as overweight and unattractive much more quickly and with fewer pounds. They are more conscious of their weight, worry about it more and consider it much more of a detriment to their happiness than men do. They are criticized for it far more than men are. And many spend a goodly portion of their waking hours preoccupied by the number of pounds they weigh.

Most women in America today are either thin or miserable because they aren't. Even a fifteen- or twenty-pound surplus is enough to make them see themselves as rejects, and many normal-sized women, with just the right amount of flesh on their bones by objective standards, think, "If *only* I could lose ten pounds." They would do much better, to our way of thinking, to accept themselves as they are, realizing that not everyone can be—or should want to be—built like a pencil. **Besides, the "ideal" weights we have become accustomed to aim for have now been acknowledged to be too low for many people to maintain realistically.** Suffering simply to be fashionable is foolish.

THE DIFFERENCES BETWEEN MEN AND WOMEN

· Men have more muscle tissue than women. Since muscle tissue burns calories faster than fat does, most men require almost double the calories to maintain a steady weight than women, who, by nature, possess a higher proportion of fat. In addition, men are usually taller and heavier with larger bones, so they require a higher expenditure of energy for any given activity. As a result, men can lose weight almost twice as fast as women on the *very same* diet and with the same amount of physical exertion.

· The average active man loses weight on as many as 2,000 to 2,200 calories a day. But the average active woman must cut back to a mere 1,000 to 1,200 to achieve the same results.

· A normal college-age man is about 15 percent fat. A twenty-year-old woman is about 25 percent fat, half of it stored just beneath the skin. By the time she is fifty-five her fat content will be about 38 percent. Women's fat usually accumulates below the waist, and, when they gain weight, they usually get thicker all over. Men, whose fat is distributed more evenly throughout their bodies, put on their excess adipose tissue mainly around their middles, backs, necks, and in a paunch that starts just over their navels.

· A man's basal metabolism rate is 6 to7 percent higher than a woman's.

· Women worry more about their weight and diet much more frequently than men. Our classes have consistently been composed of more than two-thirds women, and in commercial weight-loss groups, nine out of every ten are women. Frequently, they are not overweight at all but think they are.

· Men prefer to plan their own diet programs when they finally make the decision to lose weight. We have found that men allow themselves an average of forty to forty-five pounds over their ideal weight before they diet, while only ten or fifteen extra pounds motivates a woman. At the clinic, many women come to our classes with many fewer pounds than that to shed.

· Men are superior dieters. Not only can they lose weight faster because of their physiological advantages, but they are usually more realistic. They understand that losing weight requires eating less and exercising more, so they do it. They stay on their diets better, as soon as they see positive results. And once they have lost weight, they usually keep it off, while women tend to gain it back.

· If you ask a man why he's dieting, he will usually tell you he wants to lose weight to improve his health, his energy level or his job status. He has less need of group support while he is doing it and speculates less about *why* he is overweight and *who* is to blame.

· A woman's reasons are more internal than a man's and are tied to her self-image as well as to her relationships with other people. She wants to look younger and more attractive, improve her social life, feel more acceptable and please other people who, she is certain, will love her more when she is thin. Health, to her, is usually a peripheral issue.

· Women know far more about calories and diets and feel much more responsible for the family's health than men do. But women are much more likely to fall prey to bizarre methods of weight loss, from crash diets to drugs, plastic wraps, hypnosis and reducing machines. They will try almost anything that promises to get the weight off—fast—while admitting they *know* deep down they are falling for a hype. Most of the women in our classes have tried the same senseless fad diets numbers of times, taken pills that made them dizzy or sick, had shots of chemicals they know nothing about or spent weeks taking their meals out of bottles of liquid protein before they came to the decision to take a more sensible route. Men get there faster.

· Women are also much more likely to *over*diet, often becoming too thin for their body frames in their frenzy to be slim and fashionable. Anorexics and bulimics are almost exclusively women, usually young. Though anorexics, who starve themselves, and bulimics, who go on binges and then throw up or induce diarrhea, are fairly rare, our society abounds with women whose apparent chief interest in life is to have protruding hipbones and ribs you can count.

· Men have a better understanding of the value of exercise. They usually accept the fact that physical activity must be incorporated into a weight-loss plan. And they stay with it more faithfully once they get started. Women have more trouble squeezing regular exercise into their daily routines and give up on it a lot sooner. Fat women are major exercise haters and often will do anything short of total bed rest to avoid exerting themselves. This is unfortunate because increased exercise has a greater effect on women than on men. It increases their muscle tissue and reduces their fat. With more muscle, they can burn calories faster.

· Both men and women lie about their weight when they are fat. The heavier they are, the more they lie. (Women also like to report themselves as a little shorter than they really are, while men say they are taller.)

· Tall men, on average, reach their peak weight between the ages of thirty-five and forty-five. Shorter men (under five feet eight inches) take longer to peak. They keep gaining until they are somewhere between forty-five and fifty-four before leveling off.

· Women continue to add pounds until they are fifty-five to sixty-four years old. For them, weight jumps often correlate with pregnancies and again with menopause.

· The average adult man is five feet nine inches tall and weighs 172 pounds, while the average adult woman is slightly over five feet three and a half inches and weights 143 pounds, according to a survey by the National Center for Health Statistics.

· Spring is the most popular season for women to start diets, usually because the coming warm weather means they will have to go out without coats. But late summer or fall is the peak period for men who often relax—and expand—all summer, then find their suits are too tight.

· Men are bigger meat and starch eaters and tend to use more salt on their food. They eat less fruit, salads and greens, more fried foods. But women are more likely to be irresistibly attracted to sweets.

· A woman's disposition is more affected by her fat. She is much more apt to become depressed, irritable, discouraged because of it. Conversely, her emotions are considerably more likely, too, to be at the *root* of her weight problem. Most Compulsive Overeaters are women. They overeat because they are unhappy, bored, blue, rejected, unsuccessful, apprehensive, fearful. While some men respond to stress by overeating, most obese men get that way because of inactivity, poor nutritional habits or plain lack of concern about their bodies superimposed on a constitutional tendency to gain weight.

· Women's weight fluctuates more than men's because of their changing hormonal levels throughout the menstrual cycle. As the level of progesterone rises in relation to the amount of estrogen circulating in the bloodstream just before the menstrual period, women tend to retain water in their tissues. Some women, who do not produce high amounts of estrogen to counterbalance the progesterone, easily gain five or six more pounds in water at that time.

· Premenstrually many women have marked cravings for sweet or sometimes salty foods. Our studies of more than 1,000 women at Johns Hopkins and among flight attendants over a span of four years show that for two or three days before their periods, thin, normal and overweight women all tend to have more interest in sweets and starches. The feeling peaks on the second day of the period. But this tendency to want and to eat certain foods is much more pronounced in overweight women, and the heavier they are, the more intense the craving and the longer it lasts. The reason? Nobody knows for sure, but one promising theory is that these women have a shortage of progesterone or a drop in the level of beta endorphin and thus a reduction in the supply of serotonin, which acts as a mood elevator and appetite suppressor. Another possible cause is low blood-sugar level just before the menstrual period.

Watch out if you have this tendency to yearn for carbohydrates premenstrually because it is a simple matter to regain in one week all the weight you have lost in the previous three.*

· A diet that causes a too large or too sudden weight loss, or a diet that is continued at very low calories for too long, can interfere with a woman's menstrual cycle. Periods may vanish altogether or become shorter and lighter; they usually return to normal after healthy eating habits have been resumed.

· Women on contraceptive pills gain an average of two and a half to five pounds.

· White men tend to be fatter than black men, but black women are more frequently heavier than white women.

· Women pay the price for fat far more than men do. Our surveys find that 36 percent more derogatory comments are made about overweight women than men.

· The children in the family are likely to be feel more embar-

---

* The study of premenstrual cravings by our clinic was originated for the International Flight Attendants Association, then was expanded to include housewives, college students and industrial employees throughout the nation and abroad.

rassed about a fat mother than a fat father. However, the boys often wish their fathers could participate in sports with them.

· More men than women call a moratorium on their weight-loss diets when they go out for the evening. After all, they're out to enjoy themselves, they think, and good food is part of the fun. But more women than men order desserts in restaurants, though they may pass up the potatoes and order fish instead of meat.

· More obese males die from strokes, diabetes, accidents, kidney disease and diseases of the digestive tract than women do, while obese women have a higher incidence of cancer and cardiovascular renal disease. The danger of heart attack and angina doubles for very fat men over thin men and triples for women.

· Women have a tendency to start gaining weight after menopause for reasons no one has yet pinpointed, and the shapes of their bodies often change at the same time, losing fat around the hips, thighs and breasts and gaining it in the waistlines, rib cages and backs.

· Women are more exposed to food and therefore the temptation to eat it. As the traditional menu planners, shoppers, and cooks and the member of the family most likely to be around the house much of the time, they have as a rule more access to food and more opportunities to munch.

· Tranquilizers tend to produce a slight to moderate weight gain, especially for women. A study at our clinic showed that among the extremely overweight population, 37 percent are taking these drugs, the women outnumbering the men four to one.

· Middle-aged men frequently develop "beer bellies," protruding abdomens that rest on their belts, even though they may not have gained great amounts of weight. These are due to relaxed abdominal muscles that then develop layers of fat over them. The cure? Fewer calories and much more exercise concentrating on strengthening these muscles. For some men who can't manage to tighten this area, a girdle is the only way to avoid a hernia.

· Few very old people, men or women, are truly obese. That's because fat people die younger.

· Women tend to become thinner as they become more successful professionally. Men tend to become heavier.

5. Are You "Naturally Thin" or "Naturally Fat"? The Biological Reasons for Overweight

> My best friend eats much more than I do, especially when it comes to junk food, cookies and candy. But she is thin and I am fat. It's just not fair. I've always been told that gaining weight was a matter of too many calories, but I swear to you that everything I eat turns to fat.
>
> —Twenty-seven-year-old female secretary

Some people are "naturally thin." Others have a natural tendency to be overweight. That's why some individuals can feast with abandon and get away with it while others can't. Until recently, anyone who complained, "Everything I eat turns to fat," was accused of being a closet eater who consumed quantities of rich food when nobody was looking, a person of little self-control who could easily solve the problem by pushing away from the table. Now we know it's not that simple.

A revolutionary new concept indicates that our unique biology—not just related to gender—determines whether or not we are likely to be overweight. Though cutting calories and increasing physical activity are the only ways to reduce poundage, there is indisputable evidence today that this is *much* truer for some people than it is for others. If you discover who *you* are biologically, you will be better able to lose weight with the help you will find here from our experts.

The startling facts are:

1. **Some people gain weight and retain it much more easily than others on the very same—or maybe even fewer—calories.**

2. **Many of us were not designed by nature to be thin.**

3. The more overweight we become, and the longer we remain that way, the harder it may be to get thin and stay that way.

4. Stringent crash dieting, especially when it occurs over and over again so that the weight continually and drastically fluctuates up and down, decreases even more the ability to keep pounds off.

"SO WHAT IS THE ANSWER? DO I GIVE UP THE STRUGGLE?"

Definitely not. If you want to be thinner, you can be. But if your body holds tenaciously to its fat, you must work harder at losing it than naturally thin people do. Naturally thin people "waste" calories, burn them off easily. If you need this book, you don't. So you must keep your incoming calories at a reasonably controlled level, and even more important, you must increase your energy expenditure.

Face the facts: It may be harder for you to be thin than it is for others. But you can do it, with the help you will find here. You are not alone—millions of others have the same problem. The people who come to our weight clinic at the Johns Hopkins University are not naturally thin. Our patients are naturally overweight. But the overwhelming majority of them who stay with the program lose all or most of the weight they set out to lose and can keep it off without undue stress. *So can you.*

WHY IT'S HARDER FOR SOME PEOPLE TO BE THIN

Most overweight people do not eat more than thin people. Many actually eat less. Some individuals stay fat on a mere 1,000 calories a day; others need fewer than that. For them a "normal" diet is simply too much to handle. On the other hand, some naturally thin people can eat tremendous amounts without a big weight gain. In one scientific study, lean adult men were fed a million calories more than their normal diet in a 200-day experiment and gained very little. Why? Because they wasted them, burned them off as energy, increasing their skin temperatures and radiating the heat into the air.

If you must eat less than a normal allotment of calories in order to maintain your weight, perhaps, as one of my colleagues puts it, you are highly fuel-efficient. Instead of getting more miles to the gallon, you get more pounds to the calorie. Your body uses every incoming calorie extremely effectively, neatly storing it up inside your fat cells just in case the unlikely day arrives when you are faced by famine. Fat is the body's way of anticipating hard times.

In most cases the tendency to gain and retain weight is a genetic disposition, resulting from an inherited large or round body build with a superabundant supply of expandable fat cells. In addition, your "normal" weight—your set point—is determined by your brain, which, by automatically speeding up or slowing your ability to burn food as energy, tries to keep you just the way you are.

But fuel efficiency can also be the *consequence* of being overweight. Persistent overweight, rapid changes in weight and stringent dieting can actually change your biochemistry, slowing down your rate of metabolism so that you require fewer calories a day to *keep* you overweight than you did to *make* you overweight *originally*. That's because as you acquire more fat tissue, which takes less energy expenditure to maintain than muscle, your metabolism slows down, so you use less energy. Your body becomes a more efficient machine. And as you eat rigidly small rations, your body adjusts to less food by becoming even more efficient at burning calories. When you quit a very low-calorie diet, your body may remain at a lower metabolic rate for weeks or even months. "This energy-saving slowdown of metabolism becomes more pronounced with each weight-loss attempt," states Dr. Judith Rodin of Yale University. "It is as if the body has learned from earlier periods of deprivation and begins to slow down and decrease energy expenditures sooner and more efficiently after still another diet is begun." So it becomes increasingly more difficult to take pounds off. Life definitely is not fair!

Together these factors may erect a formidable barrier to slimming down because you must do constant battle with your own body. Research at Rockefeller University in New York has found that many obese people require a *third to a half fewer calories* to maintain their weight, pound for pound, than people with normal weight. For example, it may take 2,000 calories a day to keep one woman at 130 pounds, and only 1,200 to keep another at 350. This strange phenomenon is partially explained by the fact that fat tissue burns calories at a much lower rate than muscle does.

IS IT TRUE WHAT THEY SAY ABOUT FAT CELLS?

We all are born with our own genetic endowments of fat cells, each one of them hungry for a certain level of fat content. Some of us are born with more fat cells than average. We are the ones from families with big frames or round endomorphic bodies, or perhaps we were overnourished even before we were born.

We keep these fat cells for life. While they may shrink or expand as we lose or gain weight, they will never go away.

Turning this misdemeanor into a felony, we can increase the number of fat cells we are born with and these, too, will become permanent possessions. Two now-famous researchers, Drs. Jules Hirsch of Rockefeller University and Jerome Knittle of Mt. Sinai Medical Center in New York, confirmed a few years ago that people who start out in life as fat babies and children have abnormally large numbers of fat cells, making it probable that they will always be overweight.

If their mothers overeat, babies begin accumulating excess adipose tissue before birth. All infants experience a normal proliferation of the fat cells until the age of about a year. Knittle states that the critical periods for development of excess cells are from birth to five and again from seven to eleven. Being overweight at these times may preordain a lifetime of fighting fat.

Only a few years ago medical knowledge assumed that once childhood passed, the number of fat cells remained constant, with each cell simply expanding or shrinking depending on whether or not its owner overate. But new research indicates that even adults can produce more cells if they become very overweight. With a plethora of fat cells, there is plenty of available storage space for incoming calories.

DOES YOUR SET POINT PROGRAM YOUR WEIGHT?

Current belief is that each of us is *programmed* to be a certain weight, that we have set points, a degree of fatness at which we tend to remain, a remarkable capacity for maintaining the same body weight. Think about yourself. When you aren't paying much attention to your diet, making no conscious effort to change your weight, you probably remain within a certain few pounds. Your weight may rise a little, drop a little, but you always hover around the same mark on the scale. This is your set point.

Sometimes the set point spontaneously changes. The usual pattern is to jump up a few pounds every five years or so.

Similar to the thermostat that keeps your home's temperature constant no matter what the weather outside, the set point tends to regulate your body's fat content. There are two reasons why this may happen. It's thought, for one thing, that a regulatory mechanism in the brain senses and adjusts both appetite and energy expenditure. When your supply of fat content drops below its programmed amount and you begin to lose weight, you unconsciously desire more food. When you have returned to your set point, your appetite slacks off, and you unconsciously begin eating less.

That's not all. Your metabolism rate may alter to suit the circumstances. It automatically slows down when it gets a signal to conserve energy and speeds up to burn it, keeping your weight more or less constant. All this, the set point theory goes, applies considerable physiological pressure to stay just the way you are.

If your programmed set point suits you, be happy. But if it's set too high, so that your weight is above what you'd like, you must make changes in the way you live.

CHANGING YOUR SET POINT

What can you do if your "natural" weight is fixed too high to make you happy? You can change it. By consuming a well-balanced and nutritious low-calorie diet and by increasing your metabolic rate with exercise, you can help to *reset your set point at a lower level.*

If you are extremely overweight, you'll find that the increased physical activity is even more important than your incoming calories. This notion may put you off because exercise has never been your favorite occupation. But if you want to be thin, you must balance your energy input and outgo, and it may be impossible to cut your calories enough to make it happen without more exercise.

So be realistic. Set your goals. In this book you will find out how you can overpower your set point and get thinner.

HOW BEING FAT CAN KEEP YOU FAT

Only a very small percentage of overweight people can truthfully state that their unenviable shapes are *caused* by their hormones. But persistent overweight can affect your body chemistry. You may start out with a perfectly normal metabolism—the complex process by which food is turned into muscle, fat or energy—and end up with metabolic disturbances that interfere with your ability to keep weight off.

Indeed, one-half of all seriously overweight men and women have just such a metabolic disturbance—the vast majority as a direct consequence of having gained too much weight, according to Dr. Neil Solomon, a former colleague at the Johns Hopkins Hospital. If any of the half dozen hormones and more than 1,000 enzymes produced by the human body is not secreted in normal amounts, your metabolic rate may be slowed so much that it is almost impossible to burn enough calories to lose weight. The excess weight itself can produce the changes in your biochemistry and in your level of energy expenditure. Take your production of insulin, for example. This hormone is needed to convert blood sugar into stored fat. When you overeat, you may produce excessively high amounts of insulin, which then not only promotes fat storage rather than energy but also makes you ravenously hungry. Other hormones and enzymes are believed to act in similar ways.

This means that once you gain weight, the pounds tend to stick to your ribs. Your body becomes expert at making fat. And the longer you remain overweight, the more your metabolism may deviate from the norm. That's why it often takes fewer calories to keep you overweight than it took to get you there in the first place.

The metabolic equilibrium usually restores itself after you have lost your excess weight on a gradual balanced diet and maintained the loss. But if, instead, you put yourself through a succession of drastic freak diets, constantly gaining and losing vast numbers of pounds, you may further impair the workings of your metabolic process, making it harder and harder to reach a normal weight and stay there. So dieting itself may become the major cause of your overweight.

THE TRIPLE SOLUTION

To keep this biochemical response to its minimum, remember three things:

1. **Take weight off gradually so your metabolism doesn't respond dramatically.**

2. **Increase your exercise to help keep your BMR (basal metabolism rate) from slowing down while you diet.** Exercise also replaces fat tissue with muscle tissue, which requires more calories to exist.

3. **Never allow your weight to rise too far before going back on the program.**

HOW FAT AND THIN PEOPLE DIFFER

Here are some of the medical explanations for why overweight and thin people differ from one another:

A "Brown Fat" Deficiency.

One method of creating body heat to burn up calories is through the mechanism of brown fat. Most of our fat is white, but there are areas of dark fatty iron-containing tissue, mainly located in adults just beneath the skin around the upper back and chest and clustered near the kidneys. Rich in enzymes, which give it its color, this pigmented heat-producing fat tissue and its chemical behavior may help explain why some people can eat and get away with it and others can't.

Brown fat plays a vital part in regulating thermogenesis—internal heat production—that is not associated with the basal metabolism rate or physical activity. When an overload of calories is consumed by naturally thin people, brown fat gets to work, increasing the heat of the body so that calories are radiated into the air.

But, the theory goes, many overweight and once-overweight people do not have the capacity to turn on their thermogenesis so readily. So they collect fat instead. Researchers at the University of London make two speculations: one, that many naturally over-weight people may be endowed with *less* brown fat than naturally thin people and, two, that their brown fat may be defective in its energy-burning ability so that it does not do its assigned job efficiently.

ATPase Problem.

A related cause of the superfatted condition of some people, according to medical scientists at Harvard Medical School, is a biochemical abnormality, a deficiency of an enzyme called adenosine triphosphatase (ATPase) in the red blood cells. An estimated 10 to 50 percent of the body's heat-energy production is triggered by ATPase, which regulates sodium and potassium levels.

When too little of this enzyme circulates through the blood-stream, calories are burned less vigorously. Among the overweight subjects studied at Harvard, the ATPase level was 22 percent lower than in a control group of normal-weight volunteers. What's more, the heavier the person, the lower the enzyme level.

More research is currently under way in an effort to prove or disprove the ATPase theory.

Increased Insulin.

If you are overweight, your pancreas may turn out an abnormally high amount of insulin after you eat, and that helps keep you overweight. Insulin promotes the storage of calories in the fat cells instead of turning them into muscle tissue or energy. Besides, it makes you *hungry*. If you're already eating too much to maintain a thin body, this is obviously not helpful.

To make the situation even worse, the more calories (especially in the form of carbohydrates) eaten in a meal—and the more rapidly the food is consumed—the more insulin is released into the bloodstream. This keeps the ball rolling: You overeat, produce excess amounts of insulin, feel ravenous, eat even more, thereby releasing more insulin, which makes you hungry again.

You don't even have to eat to have insulin surge into your bloodstream, say Drs. Thomas Cooper and Judith Rodin of Yale University. Many people respond metabolically to the mere sight or smell of enticing food, even the sound of it sizzling or brewing on the stove. Sometimes just the thought of it is enough. Among a group of overweight volunteers who watched the preparation of a delectable meal, the researchers found a dramatic rise in insulin levels, far above that of normal controls.

So, while you can't literally gain weight simply by looking at food, it is true that a mere look or a listen, a whiff or a thought can turn you on physiologically so you pick up your fork and get going.

Beta Endorphin Production.

Another clue to the tendency some of us have to cling to our fat is found in recent research showing a link between overweight and circulating levels of beta endorphin, the body's natural pain-killer. Heavy people showed higher amounts of this brain opiate, which scientists theorize may stimulate appetite and reduce energy expenditure.

For Women Only—A Superabundance of Estrone.

The reason women have a higher fat content than men is that the male hormone testosterone promotes lean muscle tissue, while the female hormone estrogen's job encourages fat formation. Estrogen is produced in several forms. New research shows that while the predominant form of estrogen produced by most women during their reproductive years is estradiol, in many naturally overweight women the major form is estrone, especially adept at producing fat tissue.

According to Dr. Lila Nachtigall of the New York University Medical Center, if your estrone levels are lowered, your chances of controlling your weight are improved.

The CCK Connection.

A hormone labeled cholecystokinin (CCK), manufactured in the brain after eating, tells you when you have had enough to eat and should promptly put down your spoon.

A physician at the Bronx Veterans Administration Hospital, Dr. Rosalyn S. Yalow, won a Nobel Prize for her work with this hormone. Dr. Yalow, along with Dr. Eugene Straus, discovered that genetically obese mice have abnormally low levels of CCK in their brains and speculated that people would probably show a similar imbalance. Other scientists at the University of California in San Francisco found that the number of chemical receptors that allow CCK to enter the brain cells, turning the eating signal from green to red, significantly increased with a shortage of food and decreased with excessive food. This meant that because insufficient CCK is present when too much food is consumed by fat individuals, the proper message is not transmitted.

If the theory holds true for people, an already overweight person may continually receive the wrong signals, never feeling satisfied by perfectly adequate meals.

LPL Surplus.

Still another enzyme is involved in the problem of why weight doesn't seem to stay lost for some people. Studies at the University of Washington's General Clinical Research Center have found that the fat cells tend to hoard tryglycerides (fatty substances circulating in the bloodstream) in people who have just lost a considerable amount of weight, propelling them back to their original set points. This, say researchers, is probably caused by an overproduction of an enzyme called lipoprotein lipase (LPL) as a response to the weight loss. Among a group of obese volunteers who agreed to go on a severely restricted diet, LPL levels were three to five times higher after dieting than before. The high levels, by encouraging the fat cells to store fat, promote a quick return of the lost pounds.

PREVENTION IS THE NAME OF THE GAME

All the above biological reasons can explain why it may be hard for you to lose weight and keep it off. But before you start using the methods we have developed at our Health, Weight and Stress Program at Johns Hopkins in your search for weight loss, you must find out if you are actually overweight and, if you are, what your goal weight should be.

6. What Is Your "Best" Weight?

Americans have become so paranoid about their weight that even some slim and normal-sized people go around constantly complaining they are too fat. They talk endlessly about their waistlines, their jeans size and skim-milk cottage cheese, and for all we know, they may be just as miserable about the extra few pounds they think they have as the rest of us are about being truly overweight.

Weight consciousness is a good thing because too much fat is definitely not healthy. It can lead, as we all have been told over and over again, to diabetes, high blood pressure, aggravated arthritis, heart disease and many other hazardous health conditions we don't want to hear about anymore. **But in this country concern about weight has been carried too far.** We have become slaves to a set of "desirable weight" tables devised by the life insurance companies simply as a way to predict mortality rates, bolstered by fashion magazines and advertising, that make us feel inadequate, unattractive and unacceptable if we exceed their limits. For years we've struggled, starved and slimmed to conform to them.

GOOD NEWS AT LAST

Now deliverance! The Society of Actuaries and the Life Insurance Medical Directors of America have revised their tables, literally giving us more room for latitude. The guidelines for a "normal weight" range, so long considered gospel, have been increased by about ten pounds on average for women and fifteen to twenty pounds for men.

And new research shows that some fat isn't all that bad; in fact, a reasonable amount may even be good for you, providing emergency rations, a valuable reserve capacity that helps you survive illness.

From the National Heart, Lung and Blood Institute comes the information that the standard weight tables produce more stress for overweight Americans than inflation. The National Institutes of Health report that thin people have a higher mortality rate than people of average weight. A long-term epidemiological study in Massachusetts found that for forty- to sixty-nine-year-old women, the highest death rate was among the thinnest and the most obese, while the lowest was across a broad range of women in the intermediate-weight groups. For men, death rates *decreased* as weight went up. And an industrial study indicated that men in their fifties who were twenty-five to thirty-two percent above their "desirable" weights lived longer than *either* thinner or fatter men.

All of which demonstrates that the current standards of ideal weight used in this country definitely need revision. That's why, in our program, we recommend you take your whole self into account.

SO WHAT IS YOUR BEST WEIGHT?

The weight that's best for you depends on your body type, frame, muscular development, fat content and—most important—how you feel about your size. You should weigh an amount that makes you feel comfortable, look good, function optimally and that can be maintained without great difficulty. What is too heavy to suit one person may be just right for another, and it matters not at all if you stay within the parameters of good health. At the clinic I direct at Johns Hopkins we consider all these factors plus ethnic and cultural background, food habits and socioeconomic status as well as psychological profiles before we determine desirable weights.

Remember, choosing the best weight for you is not an exact science. In fact, there is no consensus among the experts about it. Here you will find a definition of fat, methods of measuring fat content, as well as an alternative method to the life insurance "desirable weight" tables for picking a best weight.

WHAT IS "OVERWEIGHT"? WHAT IS "OBESE"?

It's generally agreed that you are overweight if you weigh 20 percent above your "desirable" weight and that you are obese if your weight goes more than 30 percent above it. According to these standards, you are overweight if your ideal poundage is 120 and you weigh 145. And supposedly you are obese if you weigh 165.

But these numbers are not right for everyone. Since we come in assorted shapes and sizes—long-boned and narrow, square and stocky, large-boned, muscular, round, etc.—no particular number is correct for everyone of the same height and sex. Read on.

WHAT IS FAT ANYWAY?

Fat is body tissue that performs important functions. It supports and protects the internal organs, cushions the skin and manufactures antibodies to help fight disease. It insulates the body against cold, supplies a major internal source of energy and carries the fat-soluble vitamins A, E, D and K.

Fat comes in two varieties: essential and storage. Essential fat performs the jobs while the excess fat molecules from food become storage fat which settles in the fat cells waiting to be released and transformed into energy in case food supplies run low. Too much storage fat weighs down the body and slows its activity.

The average college-age man is composed of about 15 percent body fat—3 percent essential and 12 percent storage. A woman of the same age is 25 percent fat—13 percent essential and 12 per-

---

This Thing Called Cellulite

Is there such a thing as cellulite? *Cellulite* is just a fancy name somebody gave to plain ordinary fat tissue, and there is no point in treating it differently from any other kind of fat. According to Dr. Gerald Imber of the New York Hospital-Cornell Medical Center, what some people refer to as cellulite is fat that develops in little pockets. Sometimes fibrous bands develop between the fatty pockets and the skin, giving the skin a bumpy look resembling cottage cheese.

What you can do about fat, whether or not it is in pockets, is to lose weight. You cannot rid yourself of it in specific areas. Loofa sponges, pills, creams, wraps, machines, massage, special exercises and especially the diets designed to "cure cellulite" are of absolutely no value.

cent storage. A man's fat is usually dispersed fairly evenly throughout his body, while a woman's tends to be concentrated in the lower abdomen, thighs, buttocks and breasts.

Deposits of fat near the cool surfaces of the body consist chiefly of unsaturated fatty acids with a low melting point. They are actually quite watery. The deposits found internally are made up of saturated fatty acids with a high melting point. This is called hard fat, and it may be retained even on a starvation diet because it does not readily metabolize. As we grow older, our percentage of hard fat increases.

HOW MUCH OF YOU IS FAT?

Body fat is what it's all about. It is your fat content, *not* how much you weigh, that makes you overweight. So the primary criterion for true overweight is your percentage of body fat versus lean muscle mass. This means you can't totally rely on your bathroom scales to make the decision. Three women who are five feet six inches tall and weight 140 pounds can have varying amounts of body fat. One woman may be small-boned and padded with fat, one may have a large frame and be quite lean, while the third is muscular and athletic—and only the first woman could be called overweight.

A six-foot-tall football player at 250 pounds is not overweight. He is mostly muscle, with perhaps 10 percent fat content. But an office worker at the same height and weight, even the same frame, may be 35 percent fat. He is obese because his sedentary life does not make him mostly muscle.

Men normally contain less fat than women. A thin man of college age is 5 to 10 percent fat tissue. By most standards, a man with 20 percent or more fat is considered obese.

Women have more leeway when it comes to fat content because they naturally have a higher percentage of fat. Their bodies at age twenty-five are designed to be one-quarter fat. For them, 10 percent fat content is bordering on emaciation, 20 percent is thin and over 30 percent means they would be well advised to cut back their calories and step up their exercise.

As we get older, the ratio of fat tissue to muscle tissue increases for both men and women, one reason it is easier to gain weight as the years go by.

Once a Pear Shape,
Always a Pear Shape

Lose a lot of weight, and you are going to be a thinner, more attractive version of your former self, slimmer all over. But you will still possess the same general contours you started with. **Your body build and fat cell distribution never change.** In other words, if you start out *fat* and pear-shaped, you will end up *thin* and pear-shaped. If you are a short, *fat* person, you will become a short, *thin* person.

But what's so bad about that? We all are different, and that's as it should be. Some of us are naturally wide around the hips and legs; others have broad backs and square shoulders; some are straight up and down with no waistlines. And just like the color of our eyes, we are always going to retain those proportions, thin or fat.

But take heart. The fat that is the first to go when you cut calories is usually in the areas of greatest concentration. Even a tiny weight loss can make a huge difference in shape for some people. A study of women at the University of Minnesota revealed that losing as little as four pounds can cause a size change, especially if most of the weight comes off the abdomen, hips or bust. The women who were heaviest in the hips and thighs tended to lose the most in those areas, though they had to shed more weight overall to achieve a size change than those whose fat was concentrated in their upper torsos or distributed more evenly throughout their bodies.

Pear-shaped women may be happier with their configurations now that researchers at the Medical College of Wisconsin have said they are less likely to develop diabetes than women who are heavier on top. On the other hand, top-heavy women who are overweight have fewer fat cells than those with bigger bottoms, so they may find it easier to slim down.

SIZING YOURSELF UP

Before you can really know if you weigh too much, you must decide what your body frame is and then get a good idea how much of you is fat.

Body Frame.

If you've always protested, "But I have big bones!" now you can prove it. Use one of the following methods for a reasonably accurate estimate:

1. Measure your height to the nearest quarter inch. Have a friend measure the distance around your shoulders with a tape measure. Add the two numbers.

If the total is less than 99 inches, you have a small frame. From 99.1 to 106 inches, you have a medium frame. Over 106 inches means a large frame.

2. Measure the circumference of the wrist on the hand you use most.

Women: A small-boned woman will measure less than 6 inches; medium-boned, from 6 to 6½ inches. And a large-boned woman has a wrist measuring over 6½ inches.

Men: For a small frame, your wrist would measure under 6 inches. Medium frame: 6 to 7 inches. Large frame: over 7 inches.

Fat Content.

Most people use the "eyeball test" to tell them if they are too fat; you look at yourself unclothed in a full-length mirror and decide whether you like what you see. Then there's the jeans test. Do they still zip? Can you sit down in them and still breathe?

Here are two other ways to size up your situation:

1. The pinch test: Pinch yourself lightly on the back of your upper arm or your abdomen. If you find you're holding more than about an inch of yourself, you have too much fat. Women should expect a slightly thicker pinch than men because they naturally have more fat under the skin. Do not apply this test if you are over forty-five years of age because although your fat ratio increases with age, the amount found just beneath the skin diminishes.

2. Not a home method, hydrostatic weighing may be done in physiology laboratories if you are serious about determining your fat content. You are first weighed on land, then in the water on a special hydrostatic scale. Fat, being less dense than water, floats. Muscle, denser than water, sinks. The more fat you contain, the less you weigh underwater compared to your weight on terra firma.

ALTERNATIVE METHOD TO CHECK OUT "IDEAL" WEIGHT

Now that you know your body frame, try this route to finding your best weight:

Men.

Multiply your height in stocking feet by 4. Subtract 128 from the total. This number will be your "ideal" weight if you are medium-boned. If you are small-boned, subtract 10 percent. If you are large-boned, add 10 percent. For example, a large-boned man who is 73 inches tall multiplies 73 times 4, getting 292. He subtracts 128 to get 164. Now he adds 10 percent, or 16.4, for his large bones. His ideal weight is 180.4.

Women.

Multiply your height in inches by 3.5. Now subtract 108 from the total. Subtract another 10 percent for small bones, or add 10 percent for large bones. Example: If you are a medium-boned woman who is 66 inches tall, multiply 66 by 3.5 for a total of 231. Subtract 108. Your "ideal" weight is 123.

The physical aspects of your weight are of great importance in your quest to be thin because you must come to terms with your own inherited body build and your biochemical contribution to the accumulation of fat tissue. But vital, too, is your emotional investment in food, discussed in the next chapter, because it can lead you to eat more calories than your particular body can handle.

7. How Your Mind Affects Your Weight

When I'm depressed or upset about something, I start eating. I make myself a whole special meal of all the things I like, or I go to the supermarket and buy everything I know I shouldn't have in the house and go straight home and eat it. I probably think about food twenty-three hours out of every twenty-four, even when I'm sleeping. It's a good thing I'm not a drinker because I'd be an alcoholic. Food is all I think about. Eating makes me feel better until I realize what I've done.

—Middle-aged housewife

If there were simple explanations and remedies for overweight, we all would be size 8 or 42 regular. Our biological inheritance isn't the only cause of too much adipose tissue covering our bones. **Because food has such a powerful connection to our emotions, a major component of our work at the Health, Weight and Stress Program is a search for the ways people use food to fulfill their psychological needs.**

For each of us, food serves important emotional purposes. Only after these needs and responses have been identified is it possible to substitute alternative methods of satisfying them. In this chapter, with the help of our specialized techniques, you'll learn how you can look into yourself to discover your own individual ways of using food.

ANALYZING THE WAYS YOU USE FOOD

Obviously food is much more than simple sustenance. Everyone has a deep emotional investment in it. Even thin people eat—or don't eat—in response to emotions and associations. But they are luckier. They automatically burn up excess calories in energy—or know better than naturally overweight people when and how to stop spooning them in.

Overweight people, as a group, are just as well adjusted as thin people, many studies have found, and recent research indicates that—except for those who became obese in childhood—they are no more neurotic than anyone else. They do, however, suffer the emotional *effects* of being too heavy to suit the American ideal. As a result of the criticism, advice and even ridicule they receive, plus their own self-contempt, people who are far overweight often feel resentful and angry, inadequate and out of control of their own bodies. They frequently turn these feelings against themselves, making them eat even more and gain more weight.

If you are naturally thin and burn off your excess calories quickly in the production of energy, you can overeat to your heart's content, using food for comfort, distraction, release of tension or any other reason, and you won't gain much weight. Besides, you won't be criticized for it, merely observed with amazement, maybe admiration and certainly envy. But if you are naturally overweight and use food for the very same purposes, you will get fat. You won't like it, and nobody will admire you for it either.

For that reason, overweight people must find out the emotions, needs, circumstances that propel them to the candy machine or the cookie jar or that stimulate them to keep on eating long after their stomachs are full. While naturally thin people, protected by their genes, can forgo such investigation of their motives and psyches, naturally overweight people cannot. They must learn to control their impulses to eat more calories than their bodies can handle unless they are willing to settle for their "natural" weight.

A PSYCHOLOGICAL SUMMARY

It's no secret that food can be used as a tranquilizer, a pacifier, a security blanket. It provides solace, a bumper between us and reality. It helps us over the rough spots. It can comfort us when we are overwhelmed with fears and anxieties. As one of our patients told us, "I've discovered since I've been coming to the classes that I never really liked myself. I was a doormat, trying to please everybody and make them like me. I held everything in and pretended nothing was wrong. I told people, 'I don't worry about things, I'm not emotional at all.' But before I'd go to bed at night, I didn't care if I woke up the next morning. And when I got up, I started to eat and hardly stopped all day. That's changing because

I don't feel like a complete failure anymore. It shows in my weight—I've lost thirty-two pounds."

Eating food may serve as a reward for accomplishments achieved. It may be used for celebration, a way to express happiness and exuberance. In fact, in our culture, despite our over-emphasis on thinness, extravagant eating is the traditional and accepted method of noting any occasion, from birthdays to funerals to the Fourth of July.

Food can give us a temporary sense of control over the physical world around us; sometimes it seems to be the only element in our lives over which we are totally in charge. Or it can stuff a gaping inner hole of psychic emptiness, making us feel "full" instead of wanting. It can camouflage feelings of sexual inadequacy or lack of gratification. It may compensate for professional or personal shortcomings. For many of us, it is a way to relieve boredom, giving us something outside ourselves to focus upon.

Often we attempt to overcome feelings of depression or loneliness with a bag of cookies or a thick, juicy steak. And sometimes food feels like a nice comfortable bed, a haven with covers that pull up over our heads.

Some people attack their food as if it were an enemy, using it to exorcise hostility, anger, fear, resentfulness, frustration, a release for otherwise unacceptable emotions.

Others use it as a weapon to get back at other people, especially spouses or parents. As one young girl put it, "My mother always wanted me to be perfect, and she has rules for everything. She can't stand that I'm fat. She hates it. I'm a red flag waving in front of her face. Just looking at me, she knows she's failed. But I've decided I'm going to start thinking about what *I* want—and what *I* want is to be thin. If it pleases her, I can't help it!"

Psychological Insights: Mind over Matter

• The earlier the pattern of overeating begins, the quicker you lose your ability to know when and if you are physically hungry. It becomes more difficult to discriminate between hunger and anxiety.

• The person who overuses food in an attempt to relieve anxiety tends to be a person who is particularly sensitive to "pain," both physical and emotional. Compared with normal controls, overweight people as a group show more concern about their bodies and their emotional equilibrium and less tolerance for discomfort.

• Most seriously overweight people like to eat the easiest way possible and want their food readily available. An experiment at a respected university demonstrated that obese people and thin people ate differently when faced with food that was hard to get at. The thin people ate just as many nuts that were wrapped in foil as they did unwrapped nuts, while the overweight group did a much more effective job on the nuts that were easy to eat.

At our clinic, we repeated this experiment with finger foods and foods that required a knife and fork. While the thin controls ate much smaller amounts of both kinds of food than the obese group and did not differentiate between them, those who were heavy consumed three times as much finger food as the choices needing utensils.

• Overweight people are particularly sensitive to food-related environments. This helps explain why many of us lose large amounts of weight in the setting of a hospital, a weight-loss camp or a health spa but quickly revert to our former shapes and sizes soon after we return home. This is especially true of children who are sent to "fat camps."

• Once a persistently obese person starts eating, it usually takes him longer than a normal-sized person to *stop.* So, even if he doesn't eat more often, he manages to eat *more* before his brain gets the signal to quit. An experiment conducted at the University of Göttingen in West Germany demonstrated this clearly: Overweight and normal-weight subjects were fed soup through a tube, after having been told there was a certain amount of soup in the reservoir. However, the researchers continued to replenish the soup as it was consumed. The normal-weight people ate their usual portions, but the fat volunteers ate half again as much as they usually did—*even after* they had been informed about the refilling of the container.

What other uses does food serve? It may become a substitute for love and affection. It is one form of attention we can give ourselves when we don't get what we want anywhere else.

It can, by erecting a wall of fat, build a barrier between us and our responsibilities or contacts we feel we can't handle, fearing that too much would be demanded of our thinner selves. Some of us, for example, fear sexuality and what it symbolizes. Being overweight is a way to avoid confronting it or being perceived as a sex object. One young woman in our group said, "I realize now that I've been using my size so I don't have to deal with all those decisions about going to bed with somebody. I tell myself no man who isn't totally neurotic and turned on by fat women would want me. It's easier that way, but I'm working on it."

Fat makes some people feel substantial, people to be reckoned with and not overlooked as insignificant. It can symbolize power and importance.

On the other hand, for some who are afraid to compete in a social setting or in the workplace, the extra pounds provide an excuse not to take part in the race.

Some of us unconsciously use our weight as a way to gain acceptance because being fat, we pose no threat, and maybe we try to increase our welcome by becoming exceptionally helpful and willing to do the jobs nobody else wants to do.

Many people—mostly women, we have found—have a desperate need to be perfect, in total control of their destinies. Any inkling seeping into their minds that perfect control is eluding them, even momentarily, brings on an attack of eating.

For others, overeating and the consequent accumulation of fat is a form of self-punishment, a way to compensate for guilt.

And let's not neglect the people who simply love to eat, not so much because they need to satisfy deep-seated emotional needs as because they can't deny themselves anything they really want, including the pleasures of the palate.

Some of them were trained early in life to be "good children," bringing approval from their parents by eating heartily and cleaning their plates. An amazing number of our overeaters still feel in adulthood that limiting their food is a betrayal of mother and family tradition, even if Mom isn't present to exclaim over their emerging bone structures. Guilt serves the purpose.

Going on a diet is equated by some overeaters with punishment and feelings of being unloved and unacceptable.

GETTING DOWN TO CASES

What makes *you* want to eat when you know you aren't really hungry? What inner needs send you to the kitchen cupboard, the corner delicatessen or the inner recesses of your pocket, where you have stashed a chocolate bar? What makes you continue to eat even when you have consumed enough to sustain your body and you are full? Is it frustration, anger, boredom, feelings of rejection or abandonment, depression? Do you use food to bury or assuage feelings you don't want to deal with? Does eating provide comfort and familiarity? Do you feel like eating because you feel good and have reason to celebrate? Does food help satisfy you, no matter how you are feeling, up or down?

To find out whether your emotions have a strong effect on the way you eat, take this Eating Awareness Test adapted from the tests given to our patients. Your answers will give you some useful clues to your emotional investment in food by pinpointing your eating behavior.

Rate yourself, count up your score and read the evaluations following the test.

THE EATING AWARENESS TEST

How to rate yourself:

If your answer is Never, give yourself	1 point
Sometimes	2 points
Often	3 points
Very frequently	4 points
Always	5 points

Question   **Rating**

1. Do you ever say to yourself, "I've been on this diet long enough. Now I really deserve a special treat. It will make me feel better"?   _____

Question   **Rating**

2. Your hostess insists you try a second helping. Though you really shouldn't have had the first, do you have another and rationalize that you don't want to hurt her feelings?

    _____

3. When you have been craving a special treat—cream, pecan pie, chocolate—do you find you can't control it, can't hold out until the feeling dissipates?

    _____

4. When all is going well and you have just accomplished something, do you reward yourself ''just this once'' with high calories?

    _____

5. When you feel depressed, does eating raise your spirits?

    _____

6. Do you eat when you are angry, just before or just after a heated argument?

    _____

7. There's a sale on chocolate-covered caramels, doughnuts or crumb pie. Do you buy some, take it home and hide it and then eat all of it yourself?

    _____

8. When you pass your favorite candy store, gourmet food shop, bakery, are you compelled to go in and buy something?

    _____

9. No matter how hard you try, does the sight of a forbidden food get the best of you sometimes?

    _____

10. Do you deliberately eat high-calorie foods even though you don't like them?

    _____

11. Do you use food as a tranquilizer or an energy booster?

    _____

12. Do you make a ritual of eating your meals or snacks at exactly the same time every day?

    _____

13. Do you look at your empty plate and only then realize you've eaten everything on it?

    _____

14. When frustration gets the better of you, do you head for the refrigerator?

    _____

15. Do you gulp, mash, grind, slurp or inhale your food so you don't really taste it?

    _____

16. Do you prefer eating alone because no one will know what or how much you eat?

    _____

17. Have you tried many diets for brief periods of time, with partial or no long-term success?

    _____

18. Do you find that day after day you fantasize about going on a binge?

    _____

Question   **Rating**

19. Do you ever purposely plan a very rich calorie-laden meal just because you know you'll be eating alone? _____

20. Do you eat when you're not hungry? _____

21. Are you careful not to overeat when you are with others but stuff yourself when you are alone? _____

22. Do you ever feel so helpless about the way you look that you think, "What's the use?" and keep on eating? _____

23. Do you eat until you feel uncomfortable? _____

24. Do you get irresistible urges for a specific food, and would you go out even in a blizzard to get it? _____

25. Do you eat most of your food after dinner or later? _____

26. Does closet eating make you feel guilty or ashamed? _____

27. Do you hide away favorite foods to be eaten at a later time? _____

28. A tempting-looking dish has just been placed on a buffet table. You have already finished eating. Do you go ahead and eat it anyway? _____

29. Do you stock up food supplies "just in case company comes," even though you don't really need it? _____

30. Do you ever realize you haven't really tasted your food because you've covered it with condiments or eaten it too fast? _____

31. Do you eat over the sink, out of the pot, right from the refrigerator? _____

32. Are there some foods you find almost impossible to stop eating? _____

33. Do you know you eat too much but deny it when it is mentioned by other people? _____

34. Do you underestimate your caloric intake? _____

35. Are you irked when your friends or family tell you you should lose a few pounds? _____

36. Do you feel flustered and embarrassed when you're eating a large meal or a "no-no" in a public place and are spotted by someone you know? _____

37. When concentrating hard on a task, do you eat to combat mental fatigue? _____

38. Do you monitor your food intake and table manners when you are eating with others so they will think you are completely in control? _____

39. When you are reprimanded for improper food selection,

Question   **Rating**

do you stop eating it but then later eat what you want,
feeling that nobody is going to tell you what to do?   _____

40. Do you deliberately disregard your diet plan, particularly
when faced with certain foods?   _____

41. Is your family unhappy with your health or appearance?   _____

42. Do you try "miracle diets" you read about even though
you know they may not be safe?   _____

43. Do you dislike your body's appearance?   _____

44. Do you use physical complaints as an excuse for
overeating?   _____

45. Would you be ashamed if a former boyfriend (girlfriend)
or classmate showed up at a reunion and saw you as
you look now?   _____

46. Do you try on clothes you know won't fit, hoping against
hope that somehow they will look wonderful on you?   _____

47. Does being overweight make you feel inferior?   _____

48. Do you ever deliberately overeat simply because you already feel unattractive?   _____

49. Do you begin a diet thinking, "This time I'm really going
to stick to it," only to find once more you don't last more
than a week or so?   _____

50. Do you try to compensate for your size by being excessively nice and helpful to other people?   _____

51. Do you feel it is unfair that you can't eat as other people
do?   _____

52. Do you feel envious of thinner, more attractive people?   _____

53. Would you be willing to try a hazardous method of
weight reduction if it promised a rapid and remarkable
loss of pounds?   _____

54. Do you feel your size makes you unattractive to the opposite sex even when you are well dressed?   _____

55. Have you been humiliated because of a remark or ges-
ture about your weight?   _____

56. Would you pay for promises? In other words, would you
pay a high fee for a quick weight-loss method with spec-
tacular claims rather than try a more gradual proven
method?   _____

57. Do you feel being overweight makes you look older?   _____

Question   **Rating**

58. When you begin a diet, do you plan to lose more
pounds than you know you can realistically manage?   _____

59. Do you feel your weight negatively affects your sexual
desire?   _____

60. Are you very critical of other overweight people?   _____

Now add your points to get your total score.

If your score is 100 or less: Nothing for you to worry about.
When it comes to food, you have your emotions well under control. You are probably not too many pounds overweight.

101 to 145: You handle your eating behavior much better than
the average person, though occasionally you let your emotions decide what and how much you eat. You are not likely to be very
much overweight unless you have inherited a powerful tendency
toward accumulating fat. You have reasonably good insight into
your motivations. You can follow a prescribed course of action—a
diet plan—and cope with most crises well.

146 to 175: You are an average overeater. Most of the time you
can keep your eating habits under control, but often your food decisions are made on the spur of the moment without thoughtful
consideration. You tend to turn to food when things go wrong and
also when they go right. You seldom go on an all-out binge because
you come to your senses before you have gone too far.

176 to 220: Any strong feelings—and you have many of
them—can trigger you off. Your emotions control your eating behavior most of the time. Though it may occur to you that this is
happening, you convince yourself that you simply love to eat and
that good food is important to your enjoyment of life. Your insight
into your emotional problems is poor, though you may recognize
them when they are pointed out to you.

221 to 250: You have a real problem with food because you use
it to give you the strength to cope with every difficulty you encounter. You will eat anything, whether or not you like it or have
had enough. You spend much of your time thinking about what
you're going to eat for your next meal or snack. Though you think
you thoroughly enjoy good food, you really don't taste it most of
the time because you are so compulsive.

251 to 300: You have serious emotional problems about food which very likely affect your behavior in other areas, too. You are obsessive about food, using it for every possible purpose—tranquilizer, reward, compensation, self-punishment, comfort, camouflage. Your self-esteem is at the lowest possible level. You have poor insight into your feelings and the motivations for your actions. You frequently feel out of control. You are extremely tense, highly opinionated, adverse to criticism. Food means everything to you. In our opinion, you need professional help.

The Vicious Cycle of Overweight

There is a common pattern to the progression of your feelings once you become seriously overweight. If you are caught in this vicious cycle, it may be one of the reasons it's hard for you to lose weight.

The antidote to this pattern is *anticipation*. Learn to recognize the symptoms perpetuating your condition and realize they are not unique to you, so that you can interrupt the cycle. For most people, it goes something like this:

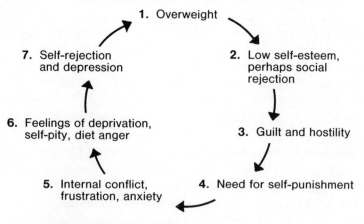

1. Overweight
2. Low self-esteem, perhaps social rejection
3. Guilt and hostility
4. Need for self-punishment
5. Internal conflict, frustration, anxiety
6. Feelings of deprivation, self-pity, diet anger
7. Self-rejection and depression

1. You become overweight.

2. Your self-esteem plummets. Perhaps you are criticized or even rejected by others.

3. As a response to your feelings of failure, you eat. You eat more than before and gain more weight. So now you are overwhelmed with guilt. Anger, resentment, hostility alienate others and further lower your sense of self-worth.

4. As payment for your "sins," you punish yourself: You stuff yourself more so that, in your own eyes, you will look worse.

5. This leads to conflict within yourself between the desire to overeat and the desire to be thin. You are frustrated because you can't make a firm decision and follow through. Anxiety and even panic may block positive moves.

6. Abstinence and deprivation in the form of extreme crash dieting or fasting seem to be the only way out for you. So you become rigid and self-disciplined—for a while. Then you start to feel sorry for yourself. Why must you suffer while other people can eat anything and get away with it?

7. You become depressed, despondent, pessimistic about your chances of ever becoming thinner. This leads to more overeating, less physical activity, and it's back to square one:

8. Overweight.

ARE YOU AFRAID TO BE THIN?

A common pattern among overweight people is to lose considerable weight and then, just as they come within striking distance of the shape they have always coveted, to panic, gaining their protective coating right back again. If this is true of you, you are actually *afraid to be thin*. It isn't that you lack will power or self-control, but you fear becoming the person you have dreamed of being, with all the expectations and responsibilities that go with it.

The fear of thinness, in fact, is so acute in some people who are afraid too much will be demanded of their thinner selves that it's actually healthier for them to stay overweight. The extra coverage serves so many psychological purposes that they cannot function well without it.

"EVERYTHING WOULD BE PERFECT IF ONLY I WERE THIN"

Overeating and overweight can give you a sense of control over your life. **You can blame all your troubles on it, thinking how**

perfect everything would be if only you were thin. Staying over-padded protects you from facing the possibility of rejection of the "real you" inside, an excuse for not meeting self-imposed or outside demands. You can continue to believe that if you become thin, you will connect with the perfect mate, find an excellent high-paying job, become irresistibly attractive and sexy, maybe get the approval you have always yearned for from your family. But you don't have to test it out, risking rejection or failure, if you stay the way you are.

The expectations of an overweight person can be enormous—and unrealistic. When you feel you can't possibly live up to them, the easiest way out may seem to be to avoid the chance of disappointment, to continue living in the fantasy world of the future when everything is going to be wonderful and you will be recognized as the great, accomplished, alluring person you really are under that comforting layer of adipose tissue.

THIN DOESN'T NECESSARILY EQUAL HAPPY

Before you even begin another weight-loss program—though this time you'll learn enough about your motivation and emotions to make success a real possibility—you must readjust your expectations. What is really likely to happen if you get thin?

Well, it will bring you better health, an improved appearance and probably more acceptance. But it's not going to make you a movie star. Men—or women—aren't going to love you exclusively for your good looks. You are probably not going to become vice-president of the company simply because of your newly acquired form, though it may help. But you've taken a step in the right direction. You will develop more self-respect, and others will find your accomplishment admirable, even though you will still be *you.* Just like everyone else, you won't be perfect and your life won't change radically unless you make it happen.

In fact, some people may try, perhaps unconsciously, to make you overeat again. Your thinness may frighten *them.* Husbands and wives have been known to worry about losing their now more attractive spouses; colleagues spot more competition from someone who was no threat before; children become concerned when Mom seems less "motherly" or Dad looks too much like a "swinger."

It takes time for everyone to adjust to your new status when you lose weight. Plan for it.

CAN YOU BE HAPPY WITH YOUR SHAPE?

Watch out. Maybe your contentment rating doesn't really depend on your fat content, but on the shape you *think* you are. Studies at our clinic clearly demonstrate that overweight and once-overweight people frequently do not know what they really look like. They have distorted body images, usually overestimating their size and the effect it has on their appearance.

Few people who have ever been very much overweight accept themselves as they are. In a survey of group members who had lost considerable weight, 65 percent considered themselves still too heavy, though only half that number were now overweight by objective standards. In fact, although they had lost even *more* than their goal amount, 11 percent of the women still felt fat.

A distorted body image—the inability to see oneself objectively—occurs in about half of the overweight population. It's particularly common among those who were obese as children or adolescents because their weight became a problem before their sense of identity and self-esteem was firmly established. Most of them *always* feel fat, no matter how thin they get.

DO YOU HAVE A "FAT HEAD"?

A major obstacle to losing weight and then staying thin is a "fat head." A thin person with a fat head is someone who always feels fat, regardless of how much he or she really weighs.

If you fit into this category, do you recognize the danger? Because you feel uncomfortable with your new status and feel it isn't really "you," you have a decided tendency to gain weight once more to reconcile the two parts of yourself. Even if you manage to remain slim, your constant fat head will make you obsessed with the numbers on your scale.

You can conquer your obstacles to contented thinness only by confronting your conflicting feelings, examining them and eventually learning to accept yourself as you are.

To find out whether your body image is distorted or real and what your feelings about your body mean to you, first take the figure-drawing test.

You will need a large sheet of paper and a sharp pencil. In no more than three minutes draw yourself as you look right now. Put your pencil down; make no more changes in the drawing. *Do not read the interpretations given below* before making your drawing.

Now ask yourself the following questions about your drawing. The interpretations of your answers should be used only as a *very rough* guide to the meaning of the picture's details. This is a simple screening test for self-evaluation only. Our tests at Johns Hopkins are evaluated by professionals and are too detailed and complicated for self-use.

1. How large is the figure? Does it take up the entire paper, half of it or only a corner? The size of the drawing is a measure of your self-confidence. If your figure fills the whole page, you are probably an assertive and forthright person who may use size as a form of power. If you have drawn a very tiny figure, perhaps you are unsure of yourself, shy and self-conscious about the way you look and relate to other people.

2. Where is the figure placed? If you drew it on the very edge of the paper, you may tend to shy away from facing facts, and you have a low estimate of yourself, a common trait among overweight people. If you drew the figure front view, you tend to be extroverted. If you drew yourself in profile, you are probably withdrawn, rigid, private and find it extremely difficult to open up about your problems, including your size. A back view can denote rejection of others, authority, or the opposite sex, as well as extreme stress. Your weight is probably one of your major problems.

3. What is the facial expression? A smile is obvious: it means an optimistic outlook, though a smile that is too intense may camouflage the opposite feeling. A turned-down mouth indicates anger, repression and a discouraged feeling about your appearance.

4. Is the head in proportion? An oversize head may indicate a predominance of reason over emotion. It may also be a sign

of self-confidence. A small head on a large body usually shows depression and inhibition along with a lack of self-confidence especially about your ability to accomplish your goals. This has an effect on your ease of losing weight.

5. How did you draw the hair? An excessive amount of hair often indicates vitality and sexuality, while too little may mean the suppression of desire, from which many overweight people suffer. No hair may mean strong inhibitions.

6. The eyes? If you drew no eyes, you tend to be out of touch with yourself and your feelings. Eyes drawn too large with overemphasized lashes may point to exaggerated responses to unrealistic goals. The nose? If it's not there or too small, you may have feelings of inferiority. The mouth? A single, straight stroke for your mouth can mean that you suppress your real desires and make too many demands on yourself. Thick, sensual lips, and a mouth that's exaggerated in size, may mean losing weight is hard for you because oral satisfaction is important to you.

7. Is your figure clothed? A naked body sometimes reflects a sense of shame about it; if it is drawn to look very fat, you are using it to punish yourself for your "ugliness." Concealing, tentlike clothes may indicate embarrassment about your body, too, and your need to hide it. Excessively detailed or frivolous garments on your figure, we have found, may mean you have unrealistic expectations about your weight and probably other aspects of your life.

8. What is the position? Clenched fists or legs wide apart denote belligerence or resentment, perhaps against dieting or authority. Legs pressed tightly together and hands behind the back may indicate sexual inhibition and/or suppressed anger.

WILL YOURSELF TO SUCCEED

Another common phenomenon among overweight people, especially women, is their readiness to *fail* at losing weight. These people don't expect to make it, so they don't. They cop out. They say, "I have no self-discipline." "I always got an F in will power." Or, "I blew it. I ate that cake; now I've ruined everything. I might as well forget it."

You will be amazed at the results you'll see if you use all the tips, tricks and suggestions we have collected at the Johns Hopkins clinic to make yourself a believer. We have seen it happen over and over again: overweight people who finally resolve to make it this time stop acting and eating like fat people.

8. Why We Like the Foods We Like

> If I could tell you all the reasons I tend to reach for a cookie instead of an apple or, better yet, my knitting, I wouldn't be in the shape I'm in today. That's why I'm in this program—to find out why I am addicted to food. I know it has to do with stress, and I've also discovered that the weather—high humidity, rain, dark skies, in particular—depress me. When I'm depressed, I turn to food.
>
> —Forty-two-year-old civil service worker

Your desire for food, the choices you make and the amount you consume are affected by many factors *outside* yourself. For example, did you know that creamy, smooth-textured foods are a favorite among the overweight, perhaps because they are unconscious reminders of home and mother, or that, if you are chronically heavy, you may be turned on to food by a bright, sunny kitchen and pink desserts?

If you sit down and make a list of the foods that really appeal to you, you will quickly discover you choose them not merely for their taste or their nourishing qualities but also because they represent something to you. They are symbolic. Perhaps they remind you of the halcyon days of your childhood, when you weren't overwhelmed with responsibilities; perhaps you associate them with celebrations, family warmth, a particular friend or occasion. Sometimes they represent comfort, security, protection against long-time discomforting feelings. Some foods are status symbols. They bolster our self-images or serve to let everyone else know who we are.

Many food preferences are, of course, learned at home. We are accustomed to them; they are part of our tradition. Others are universal favorites, even for babies. But we also *train* ourselves to like certain foods, either because they are good for us, such as fish and spinach, or because they signify "class," like strong cheeses, oysters, caviar.

In our studies of overweight people in our classes at the clinic, we have uncovered some interesting facts about food preferences. Perhaps you will recognize your own special emotional connections with what you like to eat.

DO YOU PREFER CREAMY, CRUNCHY, SPICY, EASY FOODS?

· People with serious weight problems tend, as a general rule, to prefer either (1) distinctly creamy, smooth foods or (2) those that are tough and crunchy.

Creamy foods slide down easily and take little effort to eat, so more of them can be consumed in a hurry if you are compelled to stuff yourself. "I've always felt," said one of our patients, "that if you can get food down in a hurry, it doesn't have as many calories." But most creamy, smooth foods are high in calories and appealingly sweet in flavor. Because they go down easily, the portions consumed at a sitting are usually considerably larger than comparable foods that are harder to handle.

Creamy, slippery foods often evoke childhood memories of sick days, treats, custard, ice cream, tapioca and Mom's complete and solicitous attention. They are relaxing. As one person said, "I always reach for soft foods first when I'm on a binge. I've thought about it a lot, and I know it's because I find them comforting and safe. They take me back to when life was simple and certain."

Our surveys indicate that the soft, creamy foods are most likely to be preferred by passive overeaters, people who want to please others and stay out of the fray.

On the other hand, many aggressive and angry overeaters go for tough, crunchy foods they can tear and bite, foods that "fight back." "It's like destroying the enemy," one man says. "I can chew the devil out of it. The more it snaps and cracks and resists, the better I like it."

Men are more likely to prefer foods that require vigorous attention than women who, in general, like their menus to be more accommodating.

· Hot, spicy food, as may well be expected, usually appeals most to two kinds of people: those who are feeling hot and spicy—in other words, angry—or, our surveys found, those who find life routine and unexciting and look for ways, including their food, to spice it up. Of course, spicy-food eaters also include ethnic groups that have learned to appreciate unusual flavors at the family table.

· Tolerance for unusual or difficult food textures is most limited in the morning. That's when most of us look for nourishment that "lubricates the mouth, removes the dryness of sleep, and is easily controlled and manipulated," according to an industry study. We like familiar textures in the early hours and are not so ready to accept adventures in taste then either.

· Ready-to-eat or simple-to-prepare foods are, for obvious reasons, favorites of those who tend to overeat. No fuss, no muss, just down the hatch. But we have to admit that quick foods also have special appeal to poor eaters who simply eat to live.

WHAT FOODS MAY SYMBOLIZE FOR YOU

· Meat is usually associated in our minds with strength; vegetables and fruit, with good nutrition; sweet foods, with life, happiness, fun. Red meat, according to research at Arizona State University, symbolizes "status, success, power, achievement," while sugar-laden foods represent "pleasure, self-reward and playfulness."

The researchers also found that the status seeker "who orders Indonesian roast lamb and asparagus with hollandaise sauce, washing it down with a '65 Bordeaux, is reenforcing his sense of self—and sending a message about himself to others. Doing the same is the pretty girl in bare feet and granny glasses who calls for comfrey tea with clover honey, granola and dried fruit, and carob cake."

· Again obvious, but true: Tough, chewy, pully foods attract eaters with excess nervous energy and submerged feelings of anger and insecurity. "I chew until my jaws hurt," one woman says. "I'm very impatient. I chew and do something else at the same time. It relieves my anxiety." This makes a case for chewing gum, but it is also the reason why some of us reach for the caramels instead of the soft creams or the chocolate cherries.

· Hot foods symbolize security, home, coziness, love. Has anyone's mother yet offered a cup of cold jellied madrilène when things were going awry? Hot foods stimulate us psychologically, giving a warm sense of comfort, especially when the weather is cold. Cold foods, in general, do not give off vibrations of security but may serve a purpose as reward foods—ice cream, gelatin, custard. They provide a sense of relaxation, relief, airiness, lightness.

· Overweight people, as a group, like their food to be presented attractively. For example, an experiment conducted at St. Luke's Hospital Center in New York offered in varying ways some rather tasteless liquid food to overweight and thin volunteers. The food was first given through a tube, then in a paper cup, progressed to a crystal goblet, and finally presented along with a lighted candle on a dining table.

The tube feeding discouraged the heavyweight volunteers, causing them to eat very little. The paper cup influenced them to eat twice as much as they did from the tube. The crystal goblet doubled the amount they consumed, and the candlelight increased their intake even more.

The thin subjects, however, were minimally affected by the changes.

"IT'S COLD, IT'S HOT, THE WIND IS BLOWING AND I'M HUNGRY!"

Marcia W. is a person who could be called weather-sensitive. Whenever the weather is about to change, Marcia responds by feeling depressed, irritable and disturbed. So what does she do? She eats. It makes her feel better, she says. Before she joined one of the classes in our program at Johns Hopkins, she had no idea that the fluctuations of barometric pressure, the humidity, the temperature or the amount of the sun's rays piercing the atmosphere had anything to do with her weight, and if you are weather-sensitive, you probably don't either.

But try keeping a chart, jotting down the weather and your mood, every day for about a month. **You may see a distinct correlation between your weight and weather if you are among the majority of overeaters who use food to solve your problems and soothe your spirits.**

Say the experts, it is the *change* in the weather that affects people who are most responsive, rather than the specific kinds of weather, although some people respond more to one kind of change than to another. And often the effect is felt a day or two *before* the actual alteration in weather, as a new front moves through.

About a third of the population could be termed weather-sensitive, reports Julius Fast, author of *Weather Language.* Most of them are women whose responsiveness tends to slowly rise and peak in middle-age and then to decrease.

Overweight weather-sensitive people outnumber underweights by almost two to one, according to a study made in West Germany. Do *your* unsettled weather-related feelings give you yet another incentive to have a bite to eat?

THE WEATHER AND YOUR APPETITE

Here are some other little-known facts about how what's going on in the atmosphere around you affects your weight. Many of our experiments relating to weather and appetite were based on pioneer research by Dr. Helmut Landsberg.

· Those with a tendency to be overweight gain an average of 7.43 pounds from late October until early April, our statistics at the clinic show.

· Appetites usually increase in the winter for psychological and physiological reasons. In low temperatures the body requires a higher oxygen intake to generate sufficient body heat to maintain a constant temperature. And, by raising body temperature, eating actually makes us feel warmer. Generating heat does burn off calories—if we spend time outdoors. But we tend to eat more even if we are snugly inside. Food makes us feel secure and protected from the harsh weather just outside the window.

At the same time those of us with a predisposition to be overweight and a reluctance to get out there and exercise usually get little physical activity during the winter months. What's the result of more food and less exercise? Fat.

· A drop in barometric pressure produces water retention in some people, sometimes adding as much as an inch to the circumference of a leg over a twenty-four-hour period. An increase in tissue swelling, even within the brain, can be the reason many people feel tense, depressed or irritable—with a concurrent desire to stuff themselves—when the weather changes.

· An attack of "spring fever," when it's suddenly warmer and the body shifts more blood flow to the vessels just under the skin, often makes people feel dragged out and more attracted to carbohydrates to give themselves a lift. It can correlate with a noticeable weight gain.

· Rain, our group members report, makes them eat. Why? Simply because they feel stuck in the house or the office, and eating is something to do. Rainy weather also tends to aggravate depression and anxiety, even to produce it in some sensitive people. This, in turn, makes some of us look for food.

· Weather reports of blizzards and hurricanes send hordes of shoppers to the stores to stock up on groceries. According to a nationwide survey conducted by our clinic, a high percentage of these foods tend to be sweets.

· Hot foods in cold weather warm your mouth and your fingers but don't actually raise your body temperature. Conversely, cold foods in hot weather don't cool the body. Only the *calories* in the foods affect true body heat, the same winter or summer. That's why an ice-cream cone can produce more actual body heat and energy than hot soup.

· Exercising in the winter burns more calories, if it is done out of doors in a cold temperature. It requires more energy and more effort simply to generate enough body heat. Besides, the added clothing worn in cold increases energy expenditure. That means you can lose more weight exercising when it is cold.

· Most people consume more protein in the cold months, more sweet carbohydrate foods in the warmer months.

· Less energy and therefore fewer calories are required by a normal body when temperature and humidity are high. But more fluids are essential to replace those lost in perspiration. Where dieters often go wrong in the summertime is in assuming that "light" foods are low in calories. Many of them, such as fruit juices, cold cuts, salads with oily dressings, contain plenty of calories.

· Endomorphs—shorter, rounder people—tend to be especially sensitive to warm weather and high humidity. If they respond to the weather by overeating, this factor, as well as their inherited tendency to acquire fat tissue, promotes a weight gain.

· People who live at high altitudes burn energy more quickly than those at sea level or close to it and can lose weight more easily once they make up their minds to do it.

Dieting by the Calendar

The most popular times of year for dieting are, quite logically, January or February, when many people resolve to become different people this year, and April or May, when they are desperate to look good on the beach or without a coat to camouflage the evidence.

Women are likely to start watching their weight in spring. Men prefer to begin in late summer or fall.

If we can judge the interest in weight loss by the peaks and valleys of membership in our weight-loss groups, it goes something like this: In the spring, there is a big surge of joiners, persisting until early June, when vacations begin to interfere with the best-laid plans. In early fall interest perks up once more, lasting until just before Thanksgiving. The holiday season seems to dampen enthusiasm for shaping up, but immediately after New Year's, peaking in mid-February, there is always another upsurge in resolve to slim down. Year after year, superimposed graphs of our patients show almost identical attendance patterns.

WHAT COLOR IS YOUR ARTICHOKE?

You are probably aware that the way food *looks* has much to do with whether it entices you to eat it, but **did you know you are especially turned on or off by its color? And by the colors surrounding it—for example, the plates, the tablecloth, the walls of the room?**

Perhaps these interesting facts about color and how it affects your appetite can be turned to your advantage in your efforts to slim down.

FACT: Overweight people are more affected by the appearance of their food than thin people are, and color is especially important to them. Heavy people tend to eat and drink more when their food is brightly colored than when it is pale or nondescript.

In tests in our weight classes at Johns Hopkins, the same bland, almost tasteless foods are offered in off-white and in brighter shades to groups of thin and fat people. Though the thin group's appetite for them hardly varied—they didn't like them, whatever color they were—the fat people ate far more when the color appealed to them.

FACT: About 75 percent of flavor identification of foods is based more on color than on taste, and this is particularly true for the perennially overweight. Tests with unflavored gelatin revealed, for example, that 50 percent of the time no-flavor gelatin tinted pink was judged to be cherry, raspberry or strawberry, while unflavored green gelatin was declared to be lime.

Other experiments demonstrated that when orange sherbert was colored green, 75 percent of the tasters decided it was lime. When it was tinted purple, 53 percent said it was grape. Again, more errors in identification were made by the overweight volunteers than by the thin.

FACT: "Taste" contains large components of sight and smell, a long-known fact. In our experiments, patients were blindfolded, their noses stuffed up, and they were then served their favorite foods. Most were unable to identify the foods, and many complained that the flavor was unpleasant. Of 120 subjects only 13 percent accurately named the foods.

FACT: Approximately 42 percent of our overweight members are more likely to purchase food products when they are packaged in bright colors.

FACT: In hot temperatures most people prefer foods that are green, pale yellow, pale pink, light orange or very cool tan. In cold temperatures preferences run to vivid shades like reds and oranges.

FACT: The most appealing food colors? Reds, deep peach, orange, earth tones, yellow and green (vegetables only). The least appealing? Blue and violet.

FACT: Pink desserts are the number one overall choice of overweight people.

FACT: A yellow room, a preference followed closely by warm red or orange rooms, stimulates appetite and encourages most people to eat more. But a room decorated in cool blue, green, gray or brown tends to dampen an eater's enthusiasm for food.

FACT: Dim lights depress appetites, even among dedicated

overeaters, while a brightly lit or sunny room, especially when it is decorated in sunny, warm colors, makes food seem more enticing.

FACT: Dishes affect your appetite and are a subject of intense interest in the $80-million-a-year diet business. An old behavior modification technique suggests overeaters eat from small plates with raised colored borders to give the impression of more food. Here are other helpful hints:

According to Dr. Leonard Haimes, former president of the American Society of Bariatric Physicians, you can help curb your desire to eat too much by dining from plates in quiet, pastel colors, such as pale blue, light green, pale yellow, pink, white. Shades that tend to depress appetites are grays, dark greens, dark browns, especially in solid colors.

Hues that stimulate the appetite are the warm reds, oranges, yellows, especially when they are attractively combined in bright, flowery designs.

FACT: Tablecloths, too, affect how much you eat. Food offered on white or pastel tablecloths is less appealing to hearty eaters than the same food laid out on warm, bright cloths. Red-checkered cloths, the kind you often find in Italian restaurants, especially stimulate the appetite.

FACT: A warm shade of clear rose-pink (called Baker-Miller pink) has been used in prisons and mental hospitals to decrease anxiety levels and calm aggression. The same color, applied to eight-by-ten cards and held at a comfortable distance from the eyes, tends to suppress the desire to eat for two or three hours, probably because of its relaxing influence, according to our observations of thirty participants in a study at the Johns Hopkins clinic. The volunteers were asked to concentrate on the pink card for five to thirty minutes when they felt an inordinate urge to eat. Though the results may have occurred simply through the power of suggestion, they did occur—twenty-two of the thirty reported it worked for them. One woman even painted her bedroom pink as a result!

9. Facts About Food

> I like a diet that gets the weight off fast, one I don't have to think about, just eat what it says for a couple of weeks. I've been on a lot of those diets, and they all worked; but here I am looking for another one because I'm just as fat as I ever was. I'm finding out it takes more than a diet to keep weight off me.
>
> —Forty-seven-year-old saleswoman

What you *don't* know about the food you eat can affect your health and your weight. What you *think* you know can lead you to follow ineffective, impossible-to-sustain or downright harmful diets that allow you to shed a few pounds in a hurry but not to keep them off over the long term. So, as you begin to know yourself better and learn about your unique biological and psychological reasons for overweight, for the best results you should also learn the real facts about what goes down your esophagus and into your stomach.

There are no magical foods or miraculous combinations of foods that take off weight. The only thing that takes off weight is fewer calories, consumed or burned. Your diet must provide fewer calories than you have been eating, and/or you must burn more in physical activity. Pure and simple.

But we are constantly amazed by the strange notions many otherwise intelligent dieters collect in their continuing search for slimness. For example, from new members of our classes we have heard such "facts" as: "Tomatoes clear the brain and are a good tonic for the liver, so it works better to get rid of fat"; "Lettuce helps you sleep and keeps you from waking up during the night to eat"; "Eating fat burns fat"; "You should eat very little meat when you are trying to lose weight"; "If you eat nothing but high-fiber foods, you will be healthier and thinner"; "Cheese increases the size of the bust"; "Egg whites make you retain water, and boiled eggs are thinning"; "Spinach is a diuretic"; "Nuts and sunflower seeds burn off fat"; "If you eat enough grapefruit, you can eat as much food as you want and still lose weight"; "You can lose weight by eating high-protein foods for a week, then everything you want for a week."

None of the above beliefs are true.

For a clue to your own nutritional knowledge, take the following test:

NUTRITIONAL AWARENESS TEST

Answer the question or complete each statement with *one or more* of the multiple choices.

<u>Answer</u>

1. Carbohydrates are necessary for:
   a. tissue building
   b. support of vital organs
   c. energy
          _____

2. Meat is a good source of:
   a. protein
   b. carbohydrate
   c. B vitamins
   d. calcium
          _____

3. The lowest number of calories the average man should eat per day on a reducing diet is:
   a. 1,500 to 3,000
   b. 1,200 to 1,500
   c. 3,500 to 4,000
          _____

4. The lowest number of calories the average woman should eat per day on a reducing diet is:
   a. 2,000 to 2,400
   b. 1,000 to 1,200
   c. 1,290 to 1,360
          _____

5. The average adult's daily diet should include the following amount of fluid:
   a. three glasses
   b. one glass
   c. six to eight glasses
          _____

Answer

6. For weight loss, it is best to:
 a. cut calorie intake
 b. increase physical activity
 c. fast every other day

 _____

7. In addition to citrus fruits, these foods contain high amounts of vitamin C:
 a. milk
 b. melons
 c. liver
 d. tomatoes

 _____

8. These foods are rich in protein:
 a. fruits
 b. soybeans
 c. leafy vegetables

 _____

9. Overeating cannot cause metabolic disturbances:
 a. true
 b. false

 _____

10. Vitamins are essential in a diet. When you are following a well-balanced reducing diet:
 a. vitamin supplements are necessary
 b. vitamin supplements are not necessary

 _____

11. Water is especially necessary while you lose weight because:
 a. it is a diuretic
 b. it is a source of vitamins
 c. it is needed to maintain a body chemistry balance
 d. it contains protein

 _____

12. Alcohol:
 a. contains empty calories
 b. replaces other essential foods

 _____

13. It is absolutely essential to eliminate fats from your diet in order to lose weight:
 a. true
 b. false

 _____

14. It takes the following number of calories to gain or lose a pound of weight:
    a. 1,500
    b. 2,570
    c. 3,500   _____

15. Fat cells in normal-weight and overweight people are:
    a. the same size
    b. a different size   _____

16. Who loses weight more rapidly?
    a. men
    b. women   _____

17. Who gains weight the fastest?
    a. men
    b. women   _____

18. Fasting makes your stomach shrink.
    a. true
    b. false   _____

19. The best weight-loss diet is:
    a. low in carbohydrates
    b. high in proteins
    c. all high-fiber foods
    d. none of the above   _____

20. The majority of overweight people start out with metabolic problems that cause their weight gain.
    a. true
    b. false   _____

21. When dieting, salt intake should be:
    a. increased
    b. decreased
    c. remain the same   _____

22. A typical fast-food meal includes a soft drink, french fries and a hamburger. Does this meal contain adequate protein?
    a. yes
    b. no   _____

Answer

23. An average drink (1 jigger or 1½ ounces) of 86 proof liquor contains:
    a. 50 calories
    b. 75 calories
    c. 112 calories
    d. 130 calories

_____

24. Nutrients that are likely to be inadequate in a vegetarian diet that does not include meat, fish or dairy products are:
    a. iron
    b. vitamin C
    c. vitamin A
    d. vitamin B_{12}

_____

25. Whole-wheat bread is:
    a. lower in calories than white bread
    b. higher in calories
    c. the same

_____

26. You can plan your own safe and balanced weight-loss diet accurately:
    a. if you have good nutritional knowledge
    b. if you know the number of calories you should eat per day
    c. if you take your physical activity and life-style into account

---

CORRECT ANSWERS

1. energy (c)
2. protein (a) and B vitamins (c)
3. 1,200 to 1500 (b)
4. 1,000 to 1,200 (b)
5. six to eight glasses (c)
6. cut calorie intake (a) and increase physical activity (b)
7. melons (b) and tomatoes (d)
8. soybeans (b)
9. false (b)
10. no vitamin supplements are necessary (b), unless your doctor has prescribed them for a vitamin deficiency
11. it is a diuretic (a); it is needed to maintain a body chemistry balance (b)
12. contains empty calories (a); replaces other essential foods (b)
13. false (b). The body requires a daily minimum of five grams of fat

14. 3,500 (c)

15. a different size (b). Fat cells can expand to hold more fat

16. men (a)

17. women (b)

18. false (b). Stomachs never become smaller than their normal size, though they may stretch to accommodate a large meal

19. none of the above (d). A low-calorie *balanced* diet is the best for losing and keeping weight off

20. false (b)

21. remain the same (c), unless you overuse it or have a medical condition such as high blood pressure that requires a reduction in sodium. Cutting down on salt won't help you lose fat, only water. However, most Americans routinely use too much salt.

22. yes (a), provided by the hamburger

23. 112 calories (c)

24. iron (a) and vitamin B_{12} (d)

25. the same (c)

26. (a), (b), and (c)

What Your Score Means

If you have answered all twenty-six questions correctly, you are a nutritionist, a genius, a superdieter—or you looked up the answers!

If you scored 18 to 25, you are well informed. Do you apply what you know to your own eating habits?

If you scored 15 to 17, you have average knowledge about food and its effect on your weight and health.

A score below 15 means you lack adequate information and may not get all the nutrients you need in your daily diet. You probably have tried many ineffective and perhaps unsafe weight-loss programs in the past.

WHAT DO YOU KNOW ABOUT THE FOOD YOU EAT?

Here are additional food facts to help you in your efforts to lower your weight. The more you know, the more likely you are to eat the right foods.

· Sugar is sugar, whether it is in the form of refined sugar, brown sugar, raw sugar, honey. There are little or no significant amounts of nutrients in any sugar forms including honey, and all may be called empty calories. However, except to cause tooth decay and weight gain, sugar is not harmful unless you have a problem metabolizing it or it takes the place of more nourishing food in your diet.

· Sugar comes in many disguises. Beware of any ingredients that end in *ose* or *tol.* These are usually just plain sugar. For example: dextrose, glucose, sucrose, fructose, sorbitol, mannitol, lactose. Sugar is also added to foods under other names such as corn syrup, honey, molasses. Check labels.

· Sugarless gums and candies are not calorie-free because they are sweetened with sorbitol and mannitol, which, like all carbohydrates, have a caloric value of four per gram. A stick of gum or a sugarless mint usually contains from seven to ten calories.

· There are no calories in vitamins or minerals. However, vitamins and minerals are found in the same foods that provide proteins, carbohydrates and fats.

· The foods you eat can affect both your mood and your ability to perform tasks that require concentration. Carbohydrate foods—sweets and starches—tend to raise the level of serotonin, a brain chemical that makes you more relaxed, calm, even sleepy. Proteins, on the other hand, tend to lower that level and keep you alert. A combination of both nutrients is best.

· Milk is an excellent food, if you are not allergic to it and digest it well. It is a good source of calcium especially required by older women. About a pint a day—as milk or in another form such as yogurt or cottage cheese—is a good amount to strive for. If milk causes digestive problems, try heating it or adding Lact-Aid (lactose enzyme). To keep weight and cholesterol down, use skim milk, buttermilk and low-fat milk products.

· Bananas are no more fattening than other fruits. A medium banana has about the same caloric value (100 calories) as a large orange. Bananas should be included in your diet because they provide a good source of potassium, an essential nutrient. For easy digestion, don't eat them until their skins become flecked with brown.

· Ounce for ounce, grain foods, such as bread, cereal, rice and pasta, provide fewer calories than most meats and cheeses, which contain a high proportion of fat.

· Potatoes are rich in vitamins C and B, several minerals and some protein, and they contain fewer calories than most protein

The American Eater: Part I

The average American eats 55 tons of food by the time he is seventy. This amounts to 29 tons of solid food, washed down by 6,500 gallons of liquid (of which 2,200 is coffee). It includes 9 pigs, eight cows and 15,000 eggs.

As this consumption was analyzed by a U.S. Department of Agriculture economist, the average person eats, among other foods: 1,500 pounds chicken; 1,400 pounds frankfurters, sausages, luncheon meat; 800 pounds fish; ¾ ton candy and other sweets; 6½ tons bread and grain products; 2 tons potatoes; ⅔ ton tomatoes; 600 pounds salt; 28 pounds mustard; 21 pounds pepper; 53 pounds catsup or tomato sauce; 832 pounds apples; 500 pounds bananas; 345 pounds other fruit; 1,300 gallons soft drinks; 700 gallons beer; 900 gallons tea; 900 pounds of cheese; 430 pounds butter or margarine; 3,000 pounds pasta and tacos; 4,000 pounds bread. The number of tons of refined sugar consumed per person varies in different reports.

foods. Complex carbohydrates like potatoes, bread, pasta and cereal get their bad name from what is customarily added to them in cooking or serving. In themselves they are perfect diet foods. Don't add globs of butter or sour cream, or cook them in fat. An average serving of fresh potatoes, boiled, baked or mashed with skim milk, provides about 100 calories. Half a cup of brown rice contains 90 calories. A slice of bread is about 75 calories.

On the other hand, half a cup of french fries equals about 230 calories, half a cup of fried rice has 175 and a tablespoon of sour cream adds 100 more.

Potato chips belong on nobody's diet list. They are over 40 percent fat, have few remaining vitamins or other nutrients and plenty of added salt.

· You can tell if you are eating vegetables rich in vitamin A by their color: deep green or yellow.

· Iron is essential in every diet, especially for women. High in iron are meat (especially liver), eggs, raisins, prunes, apricots, wheat germ, sardines, legumes, seeds and nuts. Lima beans are a good vegetable source. Taking some source of ascorbic acid (vitamin C) at each meal helps the absorption of the less available iron in foods.

· Fasting is never a good idea, even for a couple of days, unless you have the approval and supervision of your doctor. Prolonged fasting can cause acidosis and even death.

· Whole-grain foods have more nutrients than those made with refined grains, enriched or not.

· Fresh, frozen or canned vegetables are nutritious, though the fresh have more fiber and, if they weren't harvested too long ago, retain more vitamins. Steam fresh or frozen vegetables, or cook them briefly with as little water as possible. Cooking destroys some of the water-soluble vitamins. Don't cook canned vegetables, just heat them up.

· Canned and frozen fruits usually contain a considerable amount of sugar. Eat fresh fruit when possible. Buy water-packed canned fruits. Fruits in sugar syrup, of course, are high in calories, as are those packed in their own juice or other fruit juices.

· Fast foods are nutritionally acceptable if you have no other way to get a meal when you need it. But be discriminating. A four-ounce hamburger on half a bun is about 400 calories. Avoid the milk shakes and french fries as well as other fried foods.

· Substituting margarine for butter won't help you lose weight. Tub and bar margarine and butter all have the same caloric value—100 calories per tablespoon. So, by the way, does mayonnaise. Whipped cream cheese and whipped butter or margarine, however, have about half that amount.

· The less processed (and therefore cheaper) cereals are usually nutritionally superior to those with a long list of ingredients. Look for products with a whole grain listed as the *first* ingredient.

· Skim milk is almost fat-free. Low-fat milk contains 1 to 2 percent fat. And whole milk is about 3.5 percent fat.

· White bread has about the same caloric value as whole-wheat and other whole-grain breads, but the latter are superior nutritionally. Read the labels to be sure the main ingredient (the first one listed) is whole-grain flour. "Stoneground" whole wheat is no better than any other kind.

· Watch out for milk imitations such as nondairy creamers and fake whipped cream. They may be highly caloric, containing fat and carbohydrates as well as a long list of chemicals.

The American Eater: Part II

• An official study of the food habits of U.S. Air Force personnel reveals that, not surprisingly, overweight people prefer more meat and entrée dishes than average or underweight people. They especially like roast beef, fried shrimp, fried chicken and ham. The underweights place tossed salad among their top choices. Does this tell us something?

• The best-selling sandwiches in the United States are hamburgers and cheeseburgers, followed by ham and cheese and hot dogs. Best-selling side dish is french fries. In restaurants and other food shops, the top favorites are fried chicken, fried fish and shrimp, tuna fish, steak, roast beef, ham, chili, spaghetti, lasagna, pizza, omelets.

• Housewives today require 600 fewer calories a day than they did thirty years ago to maintain a constant weight.

• Americans' food habits are changing. Though the average weight of the U.S. population continues to increase, more people are eating foods they perceive to be light and lower in calories as well as quick and easy to prepare.

• A recent survey of our food patterns made by the U.S. Department of Agriculture and reported by the Center for Science in the Public Interest found that consumption of poultry jumped 20 percent between 1976 and 1981, while beef consumption dropped more than 19 percent, though it was compensated for by an equal increase in the amount of pork consumed. Use of low-fat milk rose 20 percent at the expense of whole milk.

• Our national consumption of soft drinks grew 25 percent in those five years, so that now Americans drink an average of 412 twelve-ounce servings a year.

• We are using more margarine and less butter, but we are consuming 34 percent more fat, 43 percent less complex carbohydrates and 45 percent more refined sweeteners than our counterparts did in 1910. Since 1976 the amount of fruits and vegetables we eat, however, has increased.

· Constipation is best overcome with high-fiber fruits, vegetables and whole grains, nuts and seeds. Especially good are figs, prunes, pears, strawberries, broccoli, cabbage, beans, celery, leafy vegetables and corn as well as all the grains and seeds.

· Whole vegetables are preferable to vegetable juices. Making juice out of them leaves most of the vegetable fiber behind as well as some carbohydrates, minerals and vitamins that are not water-soluble.

· Whole fresh fruit is preferable to fruit juice. However, fruit juices are not as nutritionally wasteful as vegetable juices. The edible portions of fruits are lower in fiber than in vegetables, and most of the nutrients are soluble in water.

· Cold cuts may give the impression of being low-calorie foods, but they are not. They are laden with fat (and salt).

· Salads also feel thin, and they are if you don't load them with rich dressings and extra toppings.

· All preservatives are not bad. Some are needed to keep food from spoiling too quickly. And even if a food is labeled "no preservatives," it does not mean no chemicals have been added. Read labels.

· It's not fattening or harmful to drink water with meals. In fact, a moderate amount of water may aid digestion and make you feel fuller as well. A bonus: If you drink a glass of water slowly ten or fifteen minutes before a meal, you will be less disposed to overeat.

· If you cook with some of the artificial sweeteners, there may be a bitter aftertaste. Add the sweetener after the food has cooled.

· Natural or "organic" foods do not have fewer calories or even an increased nutritional value, but may have fewer extraneous chemicals.

· *Fortified* means that vitamins or other nutrients are added to foods that have little or none of their own. *Enriched* means they are added to replace some of the nutrients lost in processing.

· Never substitute "fruit drinks," "juice drinks," ades or punches for fruit *juice*. Not only are they mostly water, which you can get free at home, but they are made with lots of sugar. Unsweetened juice is 100 percent fruit.

· There's no difference, except in the price, between natural and synthetic vitamins. Your body can't distinguish between a vitamin extracted from a plant or animal or produced in a laboratory.

· Just because a food is labeled "dietetic" doesn't mean it doesn't contain a lot of calories. Some contain *more* than their nondietetic counterparts, and are much more expensive besides. For example, dietetic pineapple chunks cost about twice as much as other unsweetened varieties. And dietetic, salt-free peanut butter not only has the same calories as regular peanut butter, but costs much more.

· A product labeled "diet" or "dietetic" may still contain sugar or fat, perhaps in disguised form. Or it may simply be low in salt. Check the labels.

· Don't make a practice of trying to make up for an unbalanced diet by taking vitamin pills. The best way to get all the nutrients your body needs is to eat a wide variety of foods. You need the bulk and textures of real food. Besides, food contains many nutrients in trace amounts that are not yet available in pill form.

· Dark green vegetables should be eaten when they are as fresh as possible, as all foods should be. After about five days in the refrigerator vegetables lose about half their vitamin C. Cooked vegetables lose about a quarter of their vitamin C after a day in the refrigerator, and one-third after two days. Keep frozen foods at 0 degrees or below to prevent loss of vitamins, and do not keep them too long.

· Monitor the amount of fruit juice you drink. Juices do have concentrated calories. A measuring cup of unsweetened apple juice, for example, has the same calories as two or three small apples—and less fiber.

· Learn to read labels. Federal law now requires food processors to list the ingredients on the outside of food packages, along with percentages of proteins, carbohydrates and fats. Calories are often included. If what you read sounds like something out of a high school chemistry book, try to find a similar product with fewer chemical additives.

· Water is not fattening. Because your body is about half water and you normally get rid of about three quarts a day, your health depends on replacing it. Some is replaced by food—apples, for example, are 88 percent water, and lettuce is 95 percent water—but the rest must come from drinking fluids. A normal person won't

---

The American Eater: Part III

• Overweight Americans, judged from national surveys made by our clinic at the Johns Hopkins, prefer their ice cream to be vanilla or chocolate. Strawberry is third choice. Among the sherbets, they prefer orange. Other favorite desserts: chocolate cake, cherry or strawberry pie à la mode.

• Despite protesting that they prefer "natural" foods, people often choose artificial flavors. In our tests, a highly artificial lemonade, for example, won hands down over four others, including a completely natural product, because it tasted more "lemony."

• More than half the obese people in the United States skip breakfast most of the time.

---

retain any more water than his or her body needs, so drinking water will not put on weight.

· Plain unfruited yogurt is no more fattening or thinning than milk. It is not a diet food. It contains the same number of calories as an equivalent amount of milk, whole or low-fat. When you eat yogurt with fruit (sugar is usually added) or especially with preserves, the calorie count rises astronomically.

· Toasting bread does not reduce its calories. It merely eliminates moisture.

· Puffy, airy foods are lower in calories. For example, puffed rice and puffed wheat contain only fifty-five calories per cup. Oatmeal, farina and other unsweetened hot cereals, as well as popcorn (unbuttered) and rice, can also give you considerable nourishment with remarkably few calories.

· Tempted to have a soft drink just this once? Imagine a tall glass of water with approximately eight teaspoons of sugar and a little coloring in it. Drink ice water, homemade lemonade, or iced tea with a noncaloric sweetener instead.

10. How Many Calories Should You Eat?

If you are an average woman (five feet four inches, medium frame, not too thin, not too fat), you need 1,600 to 2,400 calories a day to maintain your body weight exactly where it is, according to the National Research Council. The average man requires 2,300 to 3,000 calories a day to do the same. But each person is unique, and because your individual needs may be different, your first step in planning your new diet program is to estimate how many calories you currently are eating. Reduce this number by about 500 calories per day, and you will lose about 1 pound a week, or 52 pounds a year. Alternatively, if you eat 250 calories fewer per day and increase your exercise by 250 calories, you will also lose about 1 pound a week. If you cut out 1,000 calories a day, you will lose about 2 pounds a week. That's 104 pounds in a year!

It is never wise to eat fewer than 1,000 calories a day without close medical supervision because it is almost impossible to eat a healthy, balanced diet at such low numbers. For most people, even 1,000 are too few. If you have been consuming 2,500 to 3,000 calories a day, cutting back to 1,000 produces a weight loss that will be much too precipitous. You can't continue it for long, and the lost weight will tend to come right back to haunt you. A gradual loss is much more likely to stay lost.

FINDING OUT HOW MANY CALORIES YOU NOW EAT

Keep a Food Diary for two weeks before starting on our diet, and take a good look at what's going on when you reach for food. Though this may seem tedious at first, it is extremely important. This exercise pinpoints your trouble spots and gives you an excellent idea of your caloric intake on a typical day. You will have a detailed record of your personalized eating style and idiosyncrasies under normal circumstances.

Many people genuinely do not know how many calories they consume in a day, and many fool themselves into thinking they are cutting back when they really aren't. So, keep a record of each day's consumption so you know what you normally eat. Make a new chart for each day.

Write down exactly what you eat and drink, the method of preparation, the amount, the time, the place, the company, your hunger level, your mood, your level of stress. Do this immediately after you have eaten or even *while* you're eating. If you wait to record the information, it will be too easy to overlook some important data. Besides, you may "forget" to make entries or fail to recall your feelings at the time.

Be sure to include everything. If you picked at leftovers, write them down even if all you ate was a spoonful of corn. Be honest. Analyze your emotions and moods so you will recognize why you have eaten at that particular moment. This behavior profile will help you spot eating that is associated with specific circumstances of emotional stress.

You may find surprising revelations in your Food Diary. Perhaps you eat a perfectly normal breakfast and lunch, with very little snacking in between, but at dinner you really go at it and consume two or three portions of everything. Maybe your calories come from cocktails or from liquids—sodas, juices, lemonade, beer. Perhaps you eat more after stressful telephone conversations or when you must make a decision in your work. Are long evenings difficult for you? Maybe you undo all your good work by having a 1,000-calorie snack before you go to bed. Do you eat bread and butter before starting a meal? Your diary will tell you all.

Every night, before you go to bed, review what you have written. It's like boot camp; it's mind-training. It makes you aware of every bite you have placed in your mouth. And it can actually start you down the path to real success. We have found that in most cases overweight people start losing weight even *before* they have begun the diet because the diary makes them conscious of what, when and how they eat. It gives them unexpected insights into their eating behavior.

Make yourself a set of fourteen charts like the one following, one for each day, with space to record all meals and snacks.

After two weeks add up the approximate number of calories you consume in a typical day, using a simple calorie counter.

	Day & Date	Time	Kind & Amount of Food Eaten	Place & Circum- stances	Mood & Emotional Status	Hunger (A) & Appetite (B) Level (1 to 5)
Day 1						
Day 2						
Day 3						
Day 4						
Day 5						
Day 6						
Day 7						
Day 8						
Day 9						
Day 10						
Day 11						
Day 12						
Day 13						
Day 14						

Choose a diet plan from those in the next chapter that will provide fewer calories than you have been eating, remembering that 500 fewer calories a day add up to about a pound lost a week. Better yet, combine exercise *and* fewer calories since together they add up to *more* than the sum of the two parts.

11. The Diet That Succeeds When Others Fail

The University Medical Diet works. It is the perfect diet for people who hate to think about what they eat but have discovered that the fads are fallible. That's because it is healthy, well balanced, sensible. It's easy, it doesn't disrupt your daily life, it provides a great variety of food and it can be continued indefinitely. You can eat what you want when you want to because you choose your own food. On this diet you will safely lose one or more pounds a week—and *keep* them off. This is the intelligent person's plan, designed for those who are concerned with their health and fitness as well as with their weight.

The sample foods in this book, the explanations and the suggested menus have been developed by Gloria Elfert, M.S., R.D., and Millicent Kelly, R.D., chief nutritionists of the Johns Hopkins Hospital Department of Nutrition, based on the Exchange Lists for Meal Planning from the American Dietetic Association and the American Diabetes Association.

THE BASIC INGREDIENTS OF THE DIET

All participants in our Health, Weight and Stress Program at Johns Hopkins are interviewed by our registered dietitians, who, under the direction of Mrs. Kelly, Director of the Johns Hopkins Outpatient Nutritional Clinic, tailor a diet plan to suit each patient's individual needs and desires.

We are going to show you how to tailor your own diet, using their advice.

THE CASE FOR A BALANCED DIET

According to the hospital's nutritionists, **the calorie level of a balanced and healthy diet should include approximately 20 per-**

cent protein, 30 percent fat and 50 percent carbohydrate. This provides the nutrients needed for good body function, energy and an efficient metabolism.

Though the nutrient that overweight people can dispense with most easily is fat (because it is loaded with more than twice as many calories per gram as protein or carbohydrate), it is important to eat some of it every day. It imparts taste and palatability. More important, it provides the essential fatty acids, carries the fat-soluble vitamins the body requires, manufactures antibodies to help fight disease and is the source of long-term energy. So we suggest you cut way back on your fat intake, but be sure to include a little.

Protein, too, is a necessary component. It is used in building and repairing body tissues and regulating body processes. It provides essential nutrients, gives a feeling of satiety and helps in the metabolism of food. But protein is eaten in vastly exaggerated proportions by most Americans. Too high a percentage of protein in a low-calorie diet means you must omit other essentials needed for good health. When you eat too much protein and too little carbohydrate, there is incomplete combustion of fat and a buildup of poisonous fatty acids which may eventually result in ketosis and a serious electrolyte imbalance. Such a diet is dangerous and unhealthy if continued over a period of time, and once the diet is abandoned, weight is regained very quickly. That is why we caution against either the "quick weight-loss" high-protein diets, as well as the low-protein "diarrhea diets." Both are hazardous to your health.

The largest percentage of your daily diet should be made up of complex carbohydrates, an important source of vitamins, minerals and fiber and the primary source of energy. They should make up 50 percent—*half*—of your total daily calories. The complex carbohydrates include starches, grains, fruits, vegetables and legumes.

The University Medical Diet, as adapted by the nutritionists at Johns Hopkins, gives you a balanced, high-energy food selection in the proper proportions.

GETTING OFF TO A FLYING START

If you want to get off to a fast start, begin with the Starter Diet. This 1,000-calorie diet is balanced and complete, even though it includes significantly fewer calories than you have probably been eating. Therefore, it produces a dramatic initial weight lose. Stay on this diet one to two weeks. If your weight loss levels off at two pounds per week, continue with the same diet because this may be all the calories you can handle. If the loss exceeds two pounds a week, we strongly recommend that you abandon the Starter Diet after your flying start and choose a diet at a higher caloric level. It is not safe and not sensible to lose so rapidly.

After getting off to a fast start for its psychological value, now slow down for the long term. As we have explained, not only is quick weight loss unhealthy, perhaps even dangerous, but the weight is quickly regained. Just as important, it doesn't give you time to change your eating style and learn about your own biological and psychological attachments to fat and food so you can be realistic—and successful at last. Choose one of the diet plans offered here that give you no fewer than 1,000 calories a day less than you have been consuming. We will show you how to count up what you've been eating, then how to cut back. A thousand calories a day less then you've been consuming means a sure and steady weight loss of two pounds a week. That is the maximum you should shed over a period of time after the first week or two.

Remember, you will lose about a pound a week for each 3,500 calories you cut from your former weekly intake. That's 500 calories fewer a day. Cutting back 1,000 calories a day (7,000 per week), you will lose about two pounds. Experiment. You will soon discover what works for you.

DIET POINTERS

Here is some helpful advice for planning your diet.

1. **Do not skip meals or concentrate all (or most) of your allowed food in one or two large meals.** You will lose weight more readily with several smaller meals so your body is never overloaded at one time, then starved for available fuel at another. It is best, for your health and your weight loss, to provide your body with calories at regular intervals throughout the day.

   Maintain a regular meal schedule, spacing meals and

snacks as evenly as possible so you won't have a precipitous drop in blood sugar and hunger between them. Breakfast gets you off to a good start, especially if it includes some protein and should *never* be skipped. Researchers at the University of Texas School of Public Health in Houston recently discovered that breakfast skippers are less alert and able to solve mathematical problems in the morning than breakfast eaters. Most overweight people eat erratically and irrationally. Establish an eating routine, similar from day to day. Never feast one day and starve the next. If you prefer five or six small meals a day to three larger meals, arrange your servings accordingly.

2. **Avoid big dinners and late-night meals.** The earlier you eat, the more time your body has to digest and burn off calories in activity. Don't go to bed with a full stomach. There is some evidence that the time of day your food is consumed influences your weight. In a recent study at the University of Minnesota, people who ate 2,000 calories in one meal in the evening lost less weight than people who ate the same 2,000 in one morning. Eat a substantial breakfast and a decent lunch, and try to go easy at dinner because you are not likely to be physically active at night.

3. **Measure or weigh food after cooking it.** Foods shrink, losing water or fat in the cooking.

4. **Use a standard measuring cup** (which holds eight ounces) and measuring spoons for all foods which are portion-sized. Meat, fish and cheese may be weighed.

5. **Feel free to use any of the food choices (such as flour, bread crumbs, fat) in food preparation.** Be sure to count them in your total number of exchanges.

6. **Feel free, too, to save a fruit, bread or milk choice** from a meal menu and eat it for a snack instead.

7. **Drink six to eight glasses of fluid a day.**

8. **Forget the anticarbohydrate propaganda you've always heard.** Bread, potatoes, cereals, pasta, etc., are less fatten-

ing than most protein foods since most of the latter carry fat with them. Eat *all* your allotted starches to prevent food cravings and a lag in energy. Recent studies by researchers at the Massachusetts Institute of Technology have found that high-protein, low-carbohydrate diets produce a deficiency of an essential brain chemical called serotonin. In its effort to raise the serotonin levels, the brain may trigger almost irresistible cravings for sweets and starches, so, if you cut back drastically on carbohydrates you probably will make up for it—in spades—later on.

9. **Plan ahead.** Decide on your meals and snacks for the next week or two; then shop for what you'll need. If you don't, you will be at the mercy of your appetite and the contents of your cupboard when hunger strikes and mealtime arrives. Prepare food ahead of time, too, so it's ready when you need it.

10. **Remember, convenience foods often contain ingredients that are not on your diet** or cannot be accurately calculated. Better to avoid them for that reason and also because their availability may make them too tempting at the wrong moments.

11. **Soups, stews and combination dishes are allowed** if you prepare them with the foods allotted. Refrigerate them after cooking; then skim off the fat before reheating.

12. **Eat a wide variety of foods.** That way you won't be short on the essential nutrients that you need for good health and cannot get from pills. Besides, your menus will be more interesting and appetizing. The foods on the exchange lists contain all the vitamins, minerals and other nutrients you need. You do not need supplements unless your doctor has diagnosed a vitamin or mineral deficiency.

13. **Eat your chosen foods in the properly sized portions. Do not eat more or less** than the prescribed amounts.

14. **Plan leftovers into your menus.** For example, if you make a roast beef, use the leftovers for sandwiches or hash a few days later. None of us can afford to throw food away.

15. Though the perfect time to start the University Medical Diet program is *now*, there are some exceptions, times when it is not wise to begin a new weight-loss diet:

· During or after a severe illness, unless your doctor prescribes a weight loss and approves this diet.
· When you have been feeling depressed over a period of time.
· At the height of a major emotional crisis.

TAILORING THE DIET TO SUIT YOU

If you don't like the food on your diet, you won't be on it very long. So plan menus that make you happy. Be sure to include your favorite foods, and eliminate those you really don't like. At the clinic we conduct at Johns Hopkins, we individualize the menus for our weight group members because everyone's tastes differ. The more palatable and varied your plan is, the better you're going to enjoy it.

If you have a physical condition that requires some special diet restrictions, figure them into your choices. For example, those on low-salt diets may use fresh foods instead of canned, packaged or processed foods; fresh cucumber instead of dill pickles; and fresh ham in place of cured or smoked meats. Ask your doctor or dietitian if you have questions about what you should eat.

Important: Check out this weight-loss program with your physician. You should never go on any diet without making certain it is perfectly safe for you.

Don't be bound by tradition. Arrange your menus to suit yourself. If you feel better when you have a hearty breakfast, a medium lunch and a light supper, or if you prefer your heaviest meal at noon, go to it. Some people prefer to eat six small meals a day rather than three larger meals. This, too, is acceptable. Your daily diet will be planned by you alone.

There are only three restrictions:

· **Do not exceed the total number of calories/exchanges you have chosen to consume per day.**
· **Be sure to eat *all* your prescribed exchanges.**
· **Balance each meal as well as possible so it includes protein, fat and carbohydrate.**

MAINTENANCE: THE OLD BUGABOO

It's a fact that must be faced: **For many of us, *staying* thin is harder than *getting* thin.** The renowned Dr. Theodore B. Van Itallie, of St. Luke's Hospital Obesity Research Center in New York City, says that more people are cured of cancer than of recurring fat. **The reason is that we are willing to restrict ourselves for a certain length of time but not, heaven forbid, forever.**

Maintenance isn't the most thrilling thing that ever happened; but it can be accomplished, and it needn't mean a perpetual state of rigid control. Once you have developed insights into the way your body and emotions function in relation to food, you can learn to recognize the danger signals of a weight rebound. The most obvious one, of course, is the number of pounds you see on your scales. Never allow yourself to gain back more than three to five pounds before you return firmly to your basic diet, and take them off before they double or triple and get out of hand.

Vigilance is the key word. You cannot revert to your prediet eating habits if you want to maintain your weight loss. If you do, you will revert to your prediet shape. That is a prophecy that will definitely come true. That's why it's important to uncover the habits, attitudes, life-style, associations that led to gaining too much weight in the first place.

This is the way the participants in the weight-loss program at Johns Hopkins learn to maintain their desired weight:

1. **Lose two more pounds after you have reached your goal weight.** That gives you a little leeway for normal fluctuations and a slight gain before you catch yourself.

2. **Continue to eat the same foods you have been eating** on the weight-loss program, counting up your exchanges and watching your portions in the same way. **Then start adding a few calories.** If you have been losing about a pound a week, an addition of 350 to 500 calories should keep your weight steady. If you have been eating 1,800 calories a day, for example, and add 350 or 500, you will probably be able to eat 2,150 or 2,300 a day without gaining.

   What may be a reducing diet for one person may be a maintenance diet for another. For example, the person who loses weight on the 1,000- or 1,200-calorie diet may maintain a steady weight on the 1,500-calorie level. And the person who loses at the 1,500-calorie level may maintain on the 1,800-calorie level.

3. **Do not add the new calories suddenly.** Ease into them by giving your body just a few more calories at a time. Include about 100 more calories per day for a couple of weeks; then, if your weight holds steady at that number of calories, add another 100 a day, and so on until you have added your 350 to 500 calories without starting to gain. On the other hand, if you are still losing weight on the additional 100 calories a day, increase the amount more quickly until your weight levels off where you want it.

4. **If you find you cannot cut back or level off at enough food in your diet to make you happy and still be thin, compensate with exercise.** That will give you more latitude in calories, raise your metabolism, produce more muscle tissue which burns up more energy than fat and make you feel good besides. See Chapter 14 for the easiest ways to get more physical activity.

5. **If the pounds seem to be creeping back, you are eating too much or exercising too little, or both.** Get out your Food Diary, and start keeping note of every bite you eat. You will probably find you've been consuming more than you have been willing to admit to yourself.

6. **Be sure you have chosen a weight that is realistic,** one that you—with your unique biochemical make-up and body build, emotional composition and family background—can attain and maintain. It is far better to be a little heavier than fashion dictates—within the boundaries of good health—than to be constantly miserable. Accept yourself the way you are, even though you may not be a bag of bones. We all are, and should be, different, and there is no rational reason why we all must conform to a standard set by whoever decided we must be pencil-slim.

7. **Although maintenance may not be a simple matter** if you are naturally overweight, after a training period you can learn to adjust your calorie intake and your activity as needed quite automatically. **Use your scales to keep you alert.** Keep a weekly record of your weight near the scales

so you are always aware of it. Review the chapters on the ways your body and your mind affect your weight; retake the tests if necessary, to rediscover your unique characteristics.

8. **You have been avoiding desserts and sugary treats;** at this point be careful. Sugar is addictive—one taste and you want more. **Adding treats to your menus now is perfectly acceptable if you can control the amount you eat and keep the calories within your boundaries.** Helpful hint: If you must have a certain treat, eat it away from home. That way the remains won't be in your house to haunt you.

To illustrate graphically how different foods have different caloric values—and that calories do count—here are some numbers to contemplate:

1 cup of fat equals 2,160 calories

1 cup of sugar equals 960 calories

1 cup of spinach equals 50 calories

1 cup of water equals 0 calories

THE ALCOHOL IN YOUR LIFE

Depending on how far you must cut calories to lose weight, you needn't give up all your former habits. You don't have to go on the wagon and become a teetotaler if you can afford to pour a few extra calories in the form of alcohol into your body occasionally. Alcohol provides calories, but no other useful nutrients. An ounce of whiskey, for example, contains about 85 calories, and sweet alcoholic drinks have more.

In our program at Johns Hopkins, we do recommend that our weight-loss participants give up drinking for the duration, especially when they must cut their calories to a very low number to lose weight. But some people can lose weight at fairly high daily calorie totals, and if they can still get all the nutrition they require and spare calories for a sociable drink, we try to fit it into their diet when they really want it. We recommend light white wine because a normal portion (3½ ounces) can be worth a mere 60 to 75 calories.

Alcohol does have an effect on appetite, usually increasing it if you drink before a meal, so it's best to drink *during* your meal. And if you have it near the end of the meal, the drink may dull your desire for dessert.

Caloric Values of Alcoholic Drinks

Whiskey, scotch*	1 ounce	75–85 calories
Brandy, gin, rum, vodka*	1 ounce	75–90 calories
Liqueurs, cordials	⅔ ounce	50–80 calories
Beer, ale	8 ounces	80–150 calories
Sweet wine	3½ ounces	110–175 calories
Dry wine	3½ ounces	60–110 calories

* The higher the proof, the higher the calories.

Mixed drinks, of course, are dangerous because the added ingredients usually contain plenty of calories. Don't drink mixes such as tonic unless they are sugar-free and remember that the orange juice in a screwdriver, for example, counts toward your allotment of fruit exchanges for that day.

Here are some examples of the approximate calorie contents of mixed drinks and cocktails:

Caloric Values of Mixed Drinks

Daiquiri*	3½ ounces	134 calories
Manhattan*	3½ ounces	164 calories
Martini*	3½ ounces	140 calories
Old-fashioned	4 ounces	175 calories
Tom Collins	10 ounces	180 calories
Whiskey sour	3½ ounces	175 calories

* Commercial premixed drinks usually contain an even higher number of calories.

Reminder: Mixers are verboten because, for example, bitter lemon (10 ounces) is worth 160 calories; ginger ale and tonic (10 ounces) contain 110 calories; cola (8 ounces), 110 calories.

THE UNIVERSITY MEDICAL DIET*: HOW IT WORKS

The University Medical Diet is based on one simple idea. All approved foods are divided into six groups called Exchange Lists—milk, vegetable, fruit, bread, meat and fat—and are given caloric and nutritional ratings. Any food within a list may be exchanged for any other food on the same list, as long as it is eaten in the specified portion. That's because it is approximately equal in calories as well as in the amounts of protein, carbohydrate, fat, minerals and vitamins.

Each food, in other words, is a caloric trade-off, a nutritional equivalent of any other on the same list. You may choose what you want within each group, but you cannot trade food items from one food list to another.

The lists include hundreds of foods, everything you might ever want (with the exception of those made with concentrated sugar and fats). So you can eat normally and happily, slipping the foods you like best into your daily menus.

It's important, however, to include *all six groups* every day for a well-balanced healthy diet. Balanced nutrition means you must include daily:

- 2 milk exchanges
- 5 or 6 meat exchanges
- 3 or 4 bread exchanges
- 2 or 3 fruit exchanges (including one citrus fruit)
- 2 or 3 vegetable exchanges (including one green and one raw)
- At least 1 fat exchange

The number of exchanges depends on the number of calories in the diet plan you choose for yourself.

The first thing you need to do before beginning the diet is to decide how many calories a day you should eat if you want to lose

---

* Adapted from Exchange Lists for Meal Planning, American Diabetes Association, Inc., and the American Dietetic Association.

one or two pounds a week (500 to 1,000 calories fewer than you have been eating). Because each of us requires a different number of calories a day, the Johns Hopkins Hospital nutritionists have worked out four different food plans based on daily intakes of approximately 1,000, 1,200, 1,500 and 1,800 calories. Pick the one that suits you best.

From the six lists of foods, choose the appropriate number of exchanges for the day; then divide them into well-balanced meals and snacks. Do not eliminate any of the exchanges.

HOW TO USE THE EXCHANGE LISTS

Here are the basic rules:

1. Each food item on a list is interchangeable with any other food item on the same list—in the proper portions. For example, from the bread list, 1 slice of white bread is an exchange for ½ cup of cooked cereal, or 2 cups of plain popcorn, or 1 small white potato.

2. Foods on different lists may not be interchanged. For example, 1 slice of bread may not be exchanged for 1 portion of meat.

3. If one exchange on a food list is allowed in your plan, that means you may eat *any* item on the list in the specified amount. If two exchanges are allowed, you may take a double portion *or* two different items in single portions. For example, 2 slices of bread *or* 1 slice of bread plus ½ cup cooked cereal. Either is an allowed choice from the bread/cereals/starchy vegetables exchange list.

4. The milk and fat allowed for one day may be eaten at any meal, divided as you wish. Be sure to count them if they are used in cooking.

5. After some food items, you see notations to omit one or more fat exchanges. This means, if you include these foods—such as whole milk, corn muffins, pancakes—in your menus, you must then skip the appropriate fat exchanges. These foods already contain significant amounts of fat.

1,000-Calorie Diet (The Starter Diet)

For each day, you may eat:

2 milk exchanges
2 vegetable exchanges
3 fruit exchanges
3 bread/cereal/starchy vegetables exchanges
5 meat/fish exchanges
2 fat exchanges

1,200-Calorie Diet

For each day, you may eat:

2 milk exchanges
3 vegetable exchanges
3 fruit exchanges
5 bread/cereal/starchy vegetables exchanges
5 meat/fish exchanges
3 fat exchanges

1,500-Calorie Diet

For each day, you may eat:

2 milk exchanges
2 vegetable exchanges
5 fruit exchanges
7 bread/cereal/starchy vegetables exchanges
6 meat/fish exchanges
4 fat exchanges

1,800-Calorie Diet

For each day, you may eat:

2 milk exchanges
4 vegetable exchanges
5 fruit exchanges
7 bread/cereal/starchy vegetables exchanges
7 meat/fish exchanges
4 fat exchanges

Dividing Up Your Exchanges for One Day

You might decide to plan your meals and snacks this way, though you are free to divide your daily exchanges as you like, provided your meals are balanced and complete. You may fit snacks in where you want them, using any of the allowable foods, but try to maintain a regular eating schedule:

Sample Plans

	1,000-Calorie Diet	1,200-Calorie Diet	1,500-Calorie Diet	1,800-Calorie Diet
BREAKFAST				
Fruit exchange	1	1	1	2
Meat/fish exchange	1	1	1	2
Bread/cereals/starchy vegetables exchange	1	1	2	2
Fat exchange	1	1	1	1
Milk exchange	1	1	1	1
LUNCH				
Meat/fish exchange	2	2	2	2
Vegetable exchange	1	1	1	2
Bread/cereals/starchy vegetables exchange	1	2	2	2
Fat exchange	—	1	1	1
Fruit exchange	1	1	2	2
Milk exchange	—	—	—	—
SUPPER				
Meat/fish exchange	2	2	3	3
Vegetable exchange	1	2	1	2
Bread/cereals/starchy vegetables exchange	1	1	2	3
Fat exchange	1	1	2	2
Fruit exchange	1	1	2	2
Milk exchange	—	—	—	—
SNACK				
Bread/cereals/starchy vegetables exchange	—	1	1	1
Milk exchange	1	1	1	1

Use a form like this to plan your meals:

	Sunday	Monday	Tuesday	Wednesday	Thursday	Friday	Saturday
Breakfast							
Lunch							
Dinner							
Snack							

1. Milk Exchanges

· One exchange of skim milk contains about 12 grams of carbohydrate, 8 grams of protein, a trace of fat and 80 calories.

· Portions of each exchange vary as indicated.

· Because low-fat and whole milk contain more fat than skim milk, you must omit fat exchanges as indicated that day if you use it. We recommend only skim milk.

	Portion size
Skim or nonfat milk	1 cup
Powdered (nonfat dry, before adding liquid)	⅓ cup
Canned unsweetened evaporated skim milk	½ cup
Buttermilk made from skim milk	1 cup
Skim-milk yogurt (plain, unflavored)	1 cup
1% fat fortified milk (omit ½ fat exchange)	1 cup
2% fat fortified milk (omit 1 fat exchange)	1 cup
Yogurt made with 2% fortified milk (plain, unflavored) (omit 1 fat exchange)	1 cup
Whole milk (omit 2 fat exchanges)	1 cup
Canned evaporated whole milk (omit 2 fat exchanges)	½ cup
Buttermilk from whole milk (omit 2 fat exchanges)	1 cup
Yogurt from whole milk (plain, unflavored) (omit 2 fat exchanges)	1 cup

2. Vegetable Exchanges

· One exchange of vegetables contains about 5 grams of carbohydrate, 2 grams of protein and 25 calories.

· One exchange of the vegetables below is a ½-cup portion.

· You may eat as much as you like of the "free" raw vegetables.

· Starchy vegetables are found in the bread exchange list.

· Cook vegetables in clear water, bouillon or fat-free broth without meat or fat. Flavor them, if you like, with herbs, and seasonings as well as the fat allowed in the diet.

· Canned, fresh or plain frozen vegetables are acceptable.

Artichoke
Artichoke hearts
Asparagus
Bean sprouts
Beets
Broccoli
Brussels sprouts
Cabbage
Carrots
Cauliflower
Celery
Eggplant

Green Pepper
Greens:
  Beets
  Chards
  Collards
  Dandelion
  Kale
  Mustard
  Spinach
  Turnip
Mushrooms
Okra

Onions
Rhubarb
Rutabaga
Sauerkraut
String beans, green
  or yellow
Summer squash
Tomato juice
Tomatoes
Turnips
Vegetable juice
Zucchini

"FREE" RAW VEGETABLES

Chicory
Chinese cabbage
Chives
Cucumbers
Endive
Escarole

Lettuce
Parsley
Pickles, dill
Radishes
Scallions
Watercress

3. Fruit Exchanges

· One exchange of fruit contains about 10 grams of carbohydrate and 40 calories.

· Portions of each exchange vary as indicated.

· Cranberries may be eaten as you wish if they are prepared with noncaloric artificial sweetener.

· Fruits may be fresh, canned, unsweetened water-packed, frozen, cooked or raw, without added sugar.

· Juices must be unsweetened, taken only as a fruit choice and consumed only in the proper portions.

	Portion size
Apple	1 small
Apple juice	⅓ cup
Applesauce (unsweetened)	½ cup

	Portion size
Apricots, fresh	2 medium
Apricots, dried	4 halves
Banana	½ small
Berries	
Blackberries	½ cup
Blueberries	½ cup
Raspberries	½ cup
Strawberries	¾ cup
Cherries	10 large
Cider	⅓ cup
Cranberry juice (artificially sweetened)	¾ cup
Cranberry juice (regular)	⅛ cup
Dates	2
Figs, fresh or dried	1
Grape juice	¼ cup
Grapefruit	½
Grapefruit juice	½ cup
Grapes	12 large or 24 small
Mango	½ small
Melon	
Cantaloupe	¼ small
Honeydew	⅛ medium
Watermelon	1 slice
Nectarine	1 small
Orange	1 small
Orange juice	½ cup
Papaya	¾ cup
Peach	1 medium
Pear	1 small
Persimmon, native	1 medium
Pineapple	½ cup
Pineapple juice	⅓ cup
Plums	2 medium
Prune juice	¼ cup
Prunes	2 medium
Raisins	2 tablespoons
Tangerine	1 medium
Tomato juice	1 cup
Vegetable juice	1 cup

4. Bread/Cereals/Starchy Vegetables Exchanges

· One exchange of bread contains about 15 grams of carbohydrate, 2 grams of protein and 70 calories.

· Portions of each exchange vary as indicated.

· Note that the listed prepared foods contain significant fat, so omit fat exchanges as indicated when you include them.

· The vegetables in this group are primarily carbohydrates.

BREAD

	Portion size
Bagel, small	½
Bread sticks (nine-inch, thin)	3
Croutons	1 cup
Dried bread crumbs	3 tablespoons
English muffin, small	½
Frankfurter roll	½
Hamburger roll	½
Melba thin	2 slices
Melba toast (long)	5
Melba toast (round)	10
Pita loaf (small)	1
Raisin	1 slice
Rice cake	3
Rye or pumpernickel	1 slice
Sesame bread stick (nine-inch, large)	1
Small roll, onion, plain, seeded	1
Tortilla (six-inch)	1
White (including French and Italian)	1 slice
Whole wheat	1 slice

CEREAL

Bran flakes	½ cup
Bulgur (cooked)	½ cup
Cereal (cooked)	½ cup
Cornmeal (dry)	2 tablespoons
Cornstarch	2 tablespoons
Flour	2½ tablespoons
Grits (cooked)	½ cup

Portion size

Kasha (cooked)	½ cup
Other ready-to-eat unfrosted cereal	¾ cup
Pasta (cooked), noodles, macaroni, spaghetti	½ cup
Popcorn (popped, no fat added, large kernel)	3 cups
Popcorn (regular kernel)	2 cups
Puffed cereal (unfrosted)	1 cup
Rice or barley (cooked)	½ cup
Wheat germ	¼ cup

CRACKERS

Animal crackers	8
Arrowroot	3
Graham, 2½ inch square	2
Matzo, 4 x 6 inches	½
Oyster	20
Pretzels, 3⅛ inches long x ⅛ inch in diameter	25
Rye wafers, 2 x 3½ inches	3
Saltines	6
Soda, 2½ inches square	4
Triscuits	3
Vanilla wafers	5

DRIED BEANS, PEAS AND LENTILS

Baked beans, no pork (canned)	¼ cup
Beans, peas, lentils (dried and cooked)	½ cup

STARCHY VEGETABLES

Corn	⅓ cup
Corn on cob	1 small
Lima beans	½ cup
Parsnips	⅔ cup
Peas, green (canned or frozen)	½ cup
Potato, white	1 small
Potato (mashed)	½ cup
Pumpkin	¾ cup
Winter squash, acorn or butternut	½ cup
Yam or sweet potato	¼ cup

PREPARED FOODS

	Portion size
Biscuit, 2 inches in diameter (omit 1 fat exchange)	1
Corn bread, 2 x 2 x 1 inches (omit 1 fat exchange)	1
Corn muffin, 2 inches in diameter (omit 1 fat exchange)	1
Crackers, Ritz type (omit 1 fat exchange)	5
Muffin, plain small (omit 1 fat exchange)	1
Pancake, 5 x ½ inches (omit 1 fat exchange)	1
Waffle, 5 x ½ inches (omit 1 fat exchange)	1

5. Meat/Fish Exchanges (Includes Cheese and Eggs)

· Make most of your selections from the lists of lean and medium-fat meats. *Use the high-fat meats sparingly.*

· Portions of each exchange vary as indicated.

· All the foods listed are excellent sources of protein and other nutrients.

· Be sure to trim all visible fat from meat.

· Do not add fat or flour. If meat is fried, use only the fat included in your meal plan.

· Meat juices with fat removed may be used for added flavor.

· Measure or weigh meat *after* it has been cooked. A three-ounce serving of cooked meat is equal to about four ounces of raw meat.

· To give you a clear idea of the approximate size of a three-ounce serving of meat or fish, here are actual size illustrations of some typical choices:

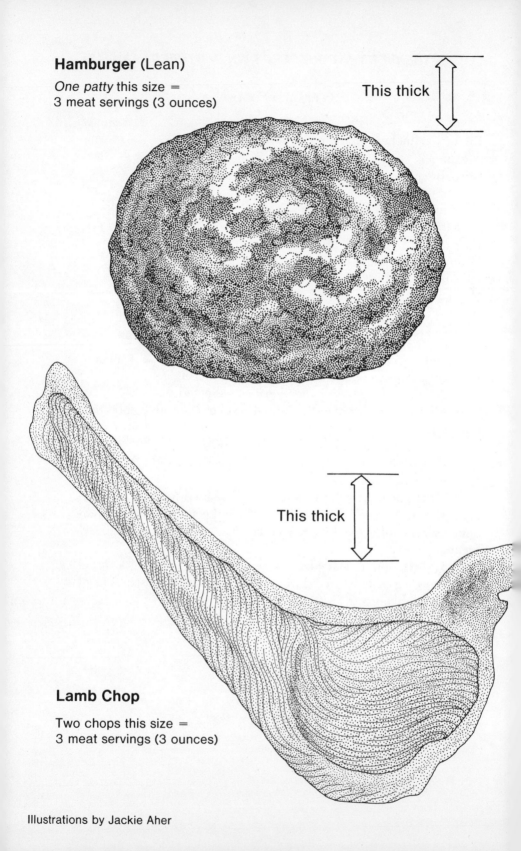

Hamburger (Lean)

One patty this size =
3 meat servings (3 ounces)

This thick

This thick

Lamb Chop

Two chops this size =
3 meat servings (3 ounces)

Illustrations by Jackie Aher

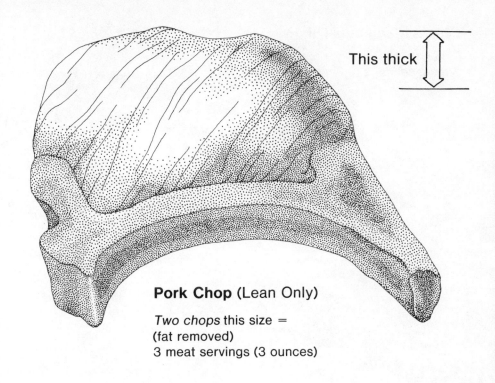

This thick

Pork Chop (Lean Only)

Two chops this size =
(fat removed)
3 meat servings (3 ounces)

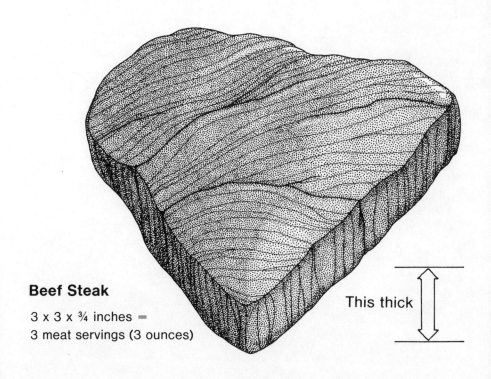

Beef Steak

3 x 3 x ¾ inches =
3 meat servings (3 ounces)

This thick

Chicken Leg and Thigh

This size =
3 meat servings (3 ounces)

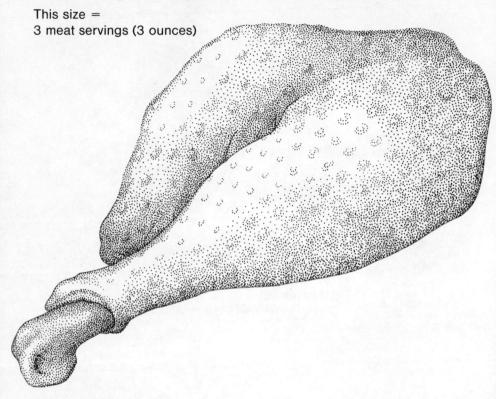

Roast Turkey

Two slices this size =
3 meat servings (3 ounces)

This thick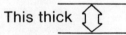

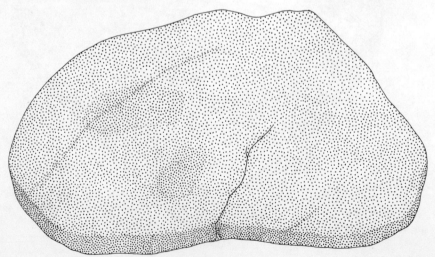

Fish

3 x 4 x¾ inches =
3 meat servings (3 ounces)

This thick

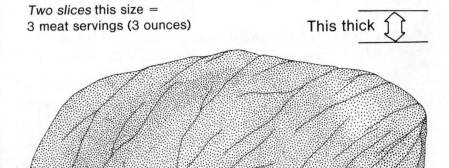

Roast Beef (Lean Only)

Two slices this size =
3 meat servings (3 ounces)

This thick

Illustrations by Jackie Aher

Lean Meat

· One exchange of lean meat contains about 7 grams of protein, 3 grams of fat and 55 calories.

Portion size

Beef:	Baby beef (very lean), chipped beef, chuck, flank steak, tenderloin, plate skirt steak, round (bottom, top), all cuts rump, spare ribs, tripe	1 ounce
Lamb:	Leg, rib, sirloin, loin (roast and chops), shank, shoulder	1 ounce
Pork:	Leg (whole rump, center shank), ham, smoked (center slices)	1 ounce
Veal:	Leg, loin, rib, shank, shoulder, cutlets	1 ounce
Poultry:	Meat (without skin) of chicken, turkey, cornish hen, guinea hen, pheasant	1 ounce
Fish:	Any fresh or frozen	1 ounce
	Canned salmon, tuna, mackerel, crab and lobster	¼ cup
	Clams, oysters, scallops, shrimp	5 or 1 ounce
	Sardines, drained	3 or 1 ounce

Low-fat cheeses (containing less than 5% butterfat)	¼ cup
Cottage cheese, dry and 2% butterfat	¼ cup
Egg substitute	¼ cup

Medium-Fat Meat

· One exchange of medium-fat meat contains about 7 grams of protein, 5 grams of fat and 75 calories.

Beef:	Ground (15% fat), canned corned beef, rib eye, round (ground commercial)	1 ounce
Pork:	Loin (all cuts tenderloin), shoulder arm (picnic), shoulder blade, Boston butt, Canadian bacon, boiled ham	1 ounce

		Portion size
Liver, heart, kidney and sweetbreads		1 ounce
Cottage cheese, creamed		¼ cup
Cheese:	Mozzarella, ricotta, farmer's cheese	1 ounce
	Neufchâtel	3 table-spoons
Egg		1

HIGH-FAT MEAT

· One exchange of high-fat meat contains about 7 grams of protein, 8 grams of fat and 100 calories
· Use sparingly.

		Portion size
Beef:	Brisket, corned beef (brisket), ground beef (more than 20% fat), hamburger (commercial), chuck (ground commercial), roasts (rib), steaks (club and rib)	1 ounce
Lamb:	Breast	1 ounce
Pork:	Spareribs, loin (back ribs), pork (ground), country-style ham, deviled ham	1 ounce
Poultry:	Capon, duck (domestic), goose	1 ounce
Veal:	Breast	1 ounce
Cold cuts:	4½ x ⅛ inches	1 slice
Frankfurter		1 small
Cheese:	Cheddar, Swiss, American, Parmesan, Gruyère, blue, Edam, Gouda, Limburger, etc.	1 ounce

6. Fat Exchanges

· One fat exchange contains about 5 grams of fat and 45 calories.
· Fats should be measured carefully because they are concentrated sources of calories.

"FREE FOODS"—TO EAT AS YOU LIKE

Artificially sweetened lemonade, iced tea

Coffee, tea, bouillon

Diet gelatin desserts

Diet soda

Dill or sour pickles*

Flavoring extracts

Free raw vegetables

Lemons and limes

Nonsugar sweeteners

Salt,* pepper, chili powder, onion salt* or powder, garlic, celery salt,* nutmeg, mint, cinnamon, mustard, paprika, other herbs and spices

* High-sodium seasonings (and pickles) must be used with caution. Try to use only a small amount, or use a salt substitute.

	Portion size
Avocado (4 inches in diameter)	⅛
Bacon	1 strip, crisp
Bacon fat	1 teaspoon
Butter	1 teaspoon
Cream, Half and Half	2 tablesoons
Cream, heavy	1 tablespoon
Cream, light	2 tablespoons
Cream, sour	2 tablespoons
Cream cheese	1 tablespoon
Lard	1 teaspoon
Margarine, diet	2 teaspoons
Margarine (regular), stick	1 teaspoon
Margarine (soft), tub or stick	1 teaspoon
Mayonnaise	1 teaspoon
Mayonnaise, imitation	2 teaspoons

DO NOT EAT

Sugar, candy, gum, jam, jelly, honey, syrup, molasses

Cookies, pies, cakes, pastries, sweet buns, puddings, diet ice cream, regular gelatin desserts

Regular soft drinks, fruit drinks, condensed milk

Cough drops, cough syrups unless prescribed or sugar-free

Catsup, chili sauce, barbecue sauce, sweet pickles

Fruits canned with juice, sugar or syrup

Deep-fried or batter-fried foods

	Portion size
Nuts	
Almonds	10 whole
Peanuts, Spanish	20 whole
Peanuts, Virginia	10 whole
Pecans	2 large whole
Walnuts	6 small
Other	6 small
Oil, corn, cottonseed, olive, peanut, saf-flower, soy, sunflower	1 teaspoon
Olives	5 small or 2 large
Salad dressing, French or Italian (regular)	1 tablespoon
Salad dressing, low-calorie	3 tablespoons
Salad dressing, mayonnaise type	2 teaspoons
Salt pork	¾-inch cube

TIPS FOR CUTTING CALORIES WHEN PREPARING FOOD

Cooking Hints

1. Before cooking meat trim off all fat with a knife or a pair of sharp scissors.

2. Before cooking poultry, remove the skin and fat.

3. Do not use self-basting birds.

4. Use lean meat in all recipes. Usually the cheaper cuts have less fat. When you buy ground beef, specify lean round or sirloin (the paler the meat, the higher the fat content), or better yet, grind your own after trimming it. Government regulations now allow 30 percent fat in ground beef. To add juiciness, grill or broil meat in beef broth when possible.

5. When pan-frying food, use a nonstick pan. Or coat the bottom of pan with a *tiny* amount of fat or spray-on coating.

6. Before cooking meat in a stew or other dish, brown it under the broiler on a rack to allow fat to drip off. If you brown it in a pan, drain off all fat before adding other ingredients.

7. Grill, broil or roast meat when possible. Use a rack to catch fat. Pour off the fat before making gravy.

8. Poach fish or poultry instead of frying it.

9. When you make soups, stew, pot roasts or meats in sauces, make them at least a day ahead, and refrigerate them. Before reheating them, remove the solidified fat.

10. Steam vegetables, or cook them in the smallest amount of bouillon or water with herbs and spices for flavor.

11. Instead of stir-frying food in oil, use water or broth, starting with a little liquid to keep it from sticking, and stir constantly, adding water as needed.

12. Always choose unsweetened juices as well as canned or frozen fruits with no sugar added.

13. Use water-packed tuna fish, or drain and rinse off the oil before eating it.

14. When broiling or baking fish, use wine, bouillon or lemon juice and other seasonings instead of butter or margarine.

15. When stuffing poultry or fish, use a vegetable stuffing or a mixture of vegetable and bread stuffings. Omit butter or oil.

16. If you use flour as a thickening agent, use it as a bread choice. Or substitute cornstarch for flour. The same amount of cornstarch has twice the thickening power of flour, and it is about equal in calories.

17. Substitute skim milk or low-fat milk for whole milk or cream.

18. Substitute low-fat yogurt for sour cream or mayonnaise.

19. Substitute low-fat cottage cheese or skim milk mozzarella for higher-calorie cheeses.

20. When meat is cooked in liquid with vegetables, as in a pot roast, refrigerate it, skim off the fat, then thicken and enrich the sauce with the puréed vegetables.

21. Use whipped butter or margarine. It contains almost half the calories of the regular bar or tub types. You can make your own whipped butter or margarine: place butter in mixing bowl; add equal part of water or skim milk; whip. Always measure fats carefully no matter what kind you use.

22. Use lemon or lime juice or vinegar on salads instead of oil.

23. Cook rice in broth, perhaps flavored with onions and green peppers. The broth (chicken, beef or vegetable) gives it enough flavor so you won't feel the need for butter. Try it, too, on vegetables. But remember, if you are on a salt-restricted diet, broth is high in sodium.

24. Learn to flavor your foods with spices and herbs, dry wines, onions, etc., so you won't want butter or sauces or gravy.

25. If bacon is on your diet, cook it *very* crisp. One strip of bacon or one teaspoon of bacon drippings equals one fat choice.

26. Rare meat often has more calories than well done, simply because more cooking releases more fat.

A WEEK OF SAMPLE MENUS

Here are sample menus for each of the four diet plans. They will demonstrate the way to divide up your calories day by day for one week. If you want to avoid food decisions temporarily, use them as they are.

SAMPLE MENUS—1,000-CALORIE DIET

SUNDAY

BREAKFAST
½ grapefruit
1 egg (or egg substitute), scrambled on nonstick pan
1 teaspoon margarine
1 slice whole-wheat toast
1 cup skim milk
Coffee or tea

LUNCH
Sandwich: 2 ounces roast turkey on 2 slices whole-wheat melba-thin bread
Lettuce and 3 slices tomato
1 wedge watermelon
Iced tea with artificial sweetener

DINNER
2 ounces broiled flounder with lemon wedge
Small baked potato with 1 tablespoon sour cream
½ cup steamed broccoli with ½ teaspoon margarine
¾ cup fresh strawberries
Tossed salad: free vegetables with Spicy Salad Dressing*

SNACK
1 cup skim milk or equivalent

* See recipes starting on p. 160.

MONDAY

BREAKFAST

½ cup orange juice

1 poached egg (or egg substitute) on ½ toasted whole-wheat
English muffin

1 teaspoon margarine

1 cup skim milk

Coffee or tea

LUNCH

Salad plate: 2 ounces water-packed tuna on lettuce bed; ½
cup asparagus spears; sliced cucumbers with vinaigrette
dressing

10 slices round melba toast

1 nectarine

Coffee or tea

DINNER

2 ounces broiled lean tenderloin

½ cup parsleyed potatoes with ½ teaspoon margarine

½ cup steamed spinach with ½ teaspoon margarine

Cucumber/radishes in vinegar, artificial sweetener

⅛ honeydew melon

Noncaloric beverage

SNACK

1 cup skim-milk chocolate junket

TUESDAY

BREAKFAST

¼ cantaloupe

1 ounce mozzarella cheese

1 small pita loaf, toasted

1 teaspoon margarine

1 cup skim milk

Coffee or tea

LUNCH

Sandwich: 2 ounces lean ham, lettuce, mustard on 2 slices rye
melba-thin bread
Dill pickle
Relish plate: ½ cup carrots, celery
1 fresh peach
Noncaloric beverage

DINNER

2-ounce broiled pork chop stuffed with ½ cup wild rice
1 teaspoon margarine
½ cup green beans
Lettuce wedge with vinaigrette dressing
Radishes
1 small baked apple
Noncaloric beverage

SNACK

1 cup skim-milk plain yogurt

WEDNESDAY

BREAKFAST

⅛ honeydew melon with lemon wedge
1 ounce grilled Canadian bacon
2 slices whole-wheat melba toast with 1 teaspoon margarine
1 cup skim milk
Coffee or tea

LUNCH

Salad plate: 10 steamed shrimp with Low-calorie Spicy Vinegar Dressing*; fresh horseradish; ½ cup sliced tomatoes on
lettuce
3 bread sticks
1 fresh pear
Noncaloric beverage

* See recipes starting on p. 160.

DINNER
2 ounces lean roast beef
½ cup steamed noodles with 2 tablespoons sour cream
½ cup cooked carrots
½ cup water-packed fruit cocktail in low-calorie Lime Gelatin*
Noncaloric beverage

SNACK
1 cup low-calorie chocolate milk shake

THURSDAY
BREAKFAST
12 grapes
1 boiled egg (or egg substitute)
½ bagel with 1 tablespoon cream cheese
1 cup skim milk
Coffee or tea

LUNCH
Open sandwich: 2-ounce broiled hamburger patty on ½ toasted hamburger roll
Kosher pickle
½ cup red beets on lettuce with low-calorie dressing
1 small apple
Noncaloric beverage

DINNER
2-ounce broiled lamb chop
½ cup green peas with 10 toasted almonds
Lettuce and tomato salad with Spicy Salad Dressing*
½ cup fresh pineapple chunks
Noncaloric beverage

SNACK
1 cup skim milk

* See recipes starting on p. 160.

FRIDAY

BREAKFAST
> 1 cup tomato juice
> ¼ cup low-fat cottage cheese
> ½ toasted whole-wheat English muffin with 1 teaspoon margarine
> 1 cup skim milk
> Coffee or tea

LUNCH
> Salad plate: ½ cup fresh crab meat on lettuce
> ½ cup coleslaw with low-calorie dressing
> 6 saltines
> 1 orange
> Noncaloric beverage

DINNER
> 2 ounces broiled rock fish
> ½ cup steamed rice
> 1 tsp. margarine
> ½ cup Creole Sauce*
> Tossed salad; free vegetables with low-calorie dressing
> ¼ cantaloupe
> Noncaloric beverage

SNACK
> 1 cup skim-milk plain yogurt

SATURDAY

BREAKFAST
> ½ cup fresh blueberries
> 1-egg (or egg substitute) omelet with 1 teaspoon margarine
> 5 slices rye melba toast
> 1 cup skim milk
> Coffee or tea

* See recipes starting on p. 160.

LUNCH
Open sandwich: 2 ounces mozzarella cheese on ½ toasted
English muffin
½ cup vegetable juice
10 Bing cherries
Noncaloric beverage

DINNER
2-ounce broiled chicken breast with unsweetened Cranberry
Sauce*
1 small car corn on the cob with 1 teaspoon margarine
½ cup coleslaw on lettuce
Cucumbers with vinegar
½ cup hot water-packed applesauce with cinnamon
Noncaloric beverage

SNACK
1 cup low-calorie vanilla milk shake

SAMPLE MENUS—1,200-CALORIE DIET

SUNDAY
BREAKFAST
¼ cantaloupe
1 slice mozzarella cheese on ½ toasted English muffin with
1 teaspoon margarine
1 cup skim milk
Coffee or tea

LUNCH
Salad plate: 2 ounces water-packed tuna; 1 teaspoon mayonnaise; ½ cup cherry tomatoes, carrot sticks, celery on lettuce
1 hard roll
1 nectarine
Noncaloric beverage

* See recipes starting on p. 160.

DINNER
2-ounce broiled lamb chop with parsley sprig
½ cup steamed rice
½ cup broccoli with lemon wedge
½ cup grated carrot with 2 tablespoons raisins, with 1 tablespoon French dressing on lettuce
Noncaloric beverage

SNACKS
1 cup skim-milk plain yogurt
2 graham crackers

MONDAY
BREAKFAST
⅛ honeydew melon with lemon wedge
1 boiled egg (or egg substitute)
1 slice whole-wheat toast
1 teaspoon margarine
1 cup skim milk
Coffee or tea

LUNCH
Sandwich: 2-ounce broiled chopped sirloin on toasted hamburger roll with mustard, dill pickle
½ cup coleslaw with 2 teaspoons mayonnaise
1 fresh pear
Noncaloric beverage

DINNER
2-ounce broiled fillet of sole with lemon wedge
Small ear of corn with ½ teaspoon margarine
½ cup coleslaw with low-calorie dressing
¾ cup fresh strawberries
Noncaloric beverage

SNACKS
1 cup skim-milk chocolate junket
5 vanilla wafers

TUESDAY

BREAKFAST

1 orange (in wedges)
1 ounce grilled Canadian bacon
½ toasted bagel with 1 tablespoon cream cheese
1 cup skim milk
Coffee or tea

LUNCH

Sandwich: 2 ounces sliced turkey breast on 2 slices whole-
  wheat bread with 1 teaspoon mayonnaise
Lettuce and tomato salad
1 wedge watermelon
Noncaloric beverage

DINNER

2 ounces broiled tenderloin
1 small baked potato with 1 tablespoon sour cream
½ cup summer squash in Creole Sauce* with ½ teaspoon
  margarine
Noncaloric beverage

SNACKS

1 cup skim milk
½ cup bran flakes

WEDNESDAY

BREAKFAST

½ cup fresh blueberries
¼ cup low-fat cottage cheese
5 slices melba toast with 1 teaspoon margarine
1 cup skim milk
Coffee or tea

LUNCH

Salad plate: ½ cup fresh crab meat; 1 teaspoon mayonnaise;
  ½ cup asparagus on lettuce with low-calorie dressing
2 sesame bread sticks
½ cup fresh pineapple
Noncaloric beverage

* See recipes starting on p. 160.

DINNER

2-ounce baked pork chop with low-calorie Barbecue Sauce*
½ cup parsleyed potatoes with ½ teaspoon margarine
½ cup steamed spinach with ½ teaspoon margarine
Tossed salad: tomatoes, mushrooms, lettuce, cucumbers and
  radishes with low-calorie dressing
1 small apple
Noncaloric beverage

SNACKS

1 cup skim-milk plain yogurt
1 cup fresh strawberries

THURSDAY

BREAKFAST

½ grapefruit
1 slice provolone cheese melted on 1 slice rye toast with
  1 teaspoon margarine
1 cup skim milk
Coffee or tea

LUNCH

Sandwich: ½ cup tomato slices and 2 ounces Swiss cheese on
  1 toasted bagel with 1 teaspoon mayonnaise and lettuce
1 small apple
Noncaloric beverage

DINNER

2 ounces roast turkey breast
½ cup baby lima beans with ½ teaspoon margarine
½ cup asparagus with ½ teaspoon margarine
½ cup red beets on lettuce with low-calorie dressing
⅛ honeydew melon
Noncaloric beverage

SNACKS

1 cup skim-milk lemon junket
3 ginger snaps

* See recipes starting on p. 160.

FRIDAY

BREAKFAST
½ banana
1 egg (or egg substitute) with 1 teaspoon margarine
¾ cup cornflakes
1 cup skim milk
Coffee or tea

LUNCH
Sandwich: 2 ounces lean roast beef on 1 toasted English muffin with fresh horseradish and mustard
Lettuce and 3 tomato slices with 1 tablespoon French dressing
1 fresh peach
Noncaloric beverage

DINNER
2 ounces roast beef
½ cup green peas with ½ teaspoon margarine
½ cup steamed cauliflower with ½ teaspoon margarine
Tossed salad with low-calorie dressing
¼ cantaloupe
Noncaloric beverage

SNACKS
1 cup skim milk
⅓ cup all-bran cereal

SATURDAY

BREAKFAST
½ cup tomato juice
1 egg (or egg substitute), scrambled in nonstick pan
1 corn muffin
1 cup skim milk
Coffee or tea

LUNCH

Salad plate: ½ cup cottage cheese on lettuce with 2 slices water-packed canned pineapple; ½ cup carrots and green peppers; 1 teaspoon mayonnaise
10 slices melba toast
Noncaloric beverage

DINNER

2 ounces barbecued chicken in low-calorie Barbecue Sauce*
½ cup potato salad on lettuce with 2 teaspoons salad dressing
½ cup coleslaw with low-calorie dressing
1 wedge watermelon
Noncaloric beverage

SNACKS

1 cup chocolate skim milk
8 animal crackers

SAMPLE MENUS—1,500-CALORIE DIET

SUNDAY

BREAKFAST

½ banana
1 cup puffed wheat
1 ounce mozzarella cheese on ½ toasted English muffin with 1 teaspoon margarine
1 cup skim milk
Coffee or tea

LUNCH

Chef's salad: 1 ounce ham, 1 ounce turkey, lettuce, cherry tomatoes; 1 tablespoon Italian dressing
24 seedless grapes
10 slices melba toast
1 nectarine
Noncaloric beverage

* See recipes starting on p. 160.

DINNER
Chicken consommé
3 ounces broiled chicken with Barbecue Sauce*
1 small baked potato with 2 tablespoons sour cream
½ cup green beans with 1 teaspoon margarine
Tossed salad: mushrooms, cherry tomatoes, green onions, celery, lettuce.
Noncaloric beverage

SNACKS
1 cup skim-milk chocolate junket
2 graham crackers

MONDAY
BREAKFAST
½ grapefruit
1 boiled egg (or egg substitute)
2 slices whole-wheat toast with 1 tablespoon cream cheese
1 cup skim milk
Coffee or tea

LUNCH
Sandwich: 2 ounces lean roast beef with horseradish and 1 teaspoon mayonnaise on hard roll
½ cup vegetable juice
1 medium apple
Noncaloric beverage

DINNER
3 ounces broiled flounder with 10 slivered, toasted almonds
1 large ear corn on the cob with ½ teaspoon margarine
1 cup broccoli, steamed with ½ teaspoon margarine, sprinkled with oregano
Sliced cucumbers in vinegar
1 wedge watermelon
Noncaloric beverage

* See recipes starting on p. 160.

SNACKS
> 1 cup skim milk
> ⅔ cup bite-size shredded wheat

TUESDAY

BREAKFAST
> ½ cup orange juice
> 1 ounce Canadian bacon
> 2 slices rye toast with 1 teaspoon margarine
> 1 cup skim milk
> Coffee or tea

LUNCH
> Salad plate: ½ cup crab meat on lettuce; 1 teaspoon mayonnaise; ½ cup asparagus spears with low-calorie dressing
> 3 rye wafers
> ½ honeydew melon
> Noncaloric beverage

DINNER
> Beef consommé
> 3 1-ounce meat balls with 1 cup spaghetti sauce and ½ cup spaghetti
> 1 slice French bread, toasted, with 1 teaspoon margarine
> Tossed salad with 1 tablespoon Italian dressing
> ¼ cantaloupe
> Noncaloric beverage

SNACKS
> 1 cup skim-milk plain yogurt
> 1 sesame bread stick

WEDNESDAY

BREAKFAST
> ½ cup fresh blueberries
> ¾ cup corn flakes
> 1 egg (or egg substitute), scrambled on nonstick pan
> 1 small corn muffin, toasted
> 1 cup skim milk
> Coffee or tea

LUNCH

Sandwich: 2 ounces roasted chicken on 2 slices rye bread, toasted, with 1 teaspoon mayonnaise, lettuce

Relish plate: carrots, celery, dill pickle

1 cup orange and grapefruit sections

Noncaloric beverage

DINNER

Beef kabobs: 3 ounces sirloin tip, cut into 1½-inch cubes, marinated in Barbecue Sauce* with added soy sauce

½ cup cherry tomatoes, small onions, green pepper

½ cup steamed rice with 1 teaspoon margarine and saffron

½ cup vegetable juice

½ cup fresh pineapple chunks

1 cornmeal muffin

Noncaloric beverage

SNACKS

1 cup skim-milk vanilla junket

5 slices melba toast

THURSDAY

BREAKFAST

⅛ honeydew melon

1 ounce smoked salmon

1 whole-wheat or rye bagel with 1 tablespoon cream cheese

1 cup skim milk

Coffee or tea

LUNCH

Salad plate: ½ cup low-fat cottage cheese on lettuce; 1 fresh peach; 24 seedless grapes

½ cup tomato juice

10 slices melba toast

Iced tea with lemon

* See recipes starting on p. 160.

DINNER

3 ounces broiled lobster tails with 1 teaspoon margarine
1 large baked potato with 2 tablespoons sour cream
1 cup zucchini with Creole Sauce*
Lettuce wedge with low-calorie dressing
¾ cup fresh strawberries
Noncaloric beverage

SNACKS

1 cup skim milk
½ cup raisin bran

FRIDAY

BREAKFAST

¼ cantaloupe
¼ cup low-fat cottage cheese with 1 tablespoon cream cheese, melted on 2 slices raisin toast, sprinkled with nutmeg and cinnamon
1 cup low-calorie cocoa
Coffee or tea

LUNCH

Sandwich: 2-ounce broiled hamburger patty on toasted hamburger roll with mustard, lettuce, tomato, 1 teaspoon mayonnaise
1 banana
Noncaloric beverage

DINNER

3 ounces roast beef
1 cup cooked noodles with 2 tablespoon sour cream
½ cup cooked carrots with mint sprig
Lettuce and tomato salad with low-calorie dressing
10 cherries
Noncaloric beverage

SNACKS

1 cup skim-milk plain yogurt
1 cup fresh strawberries

* See recipes starting on p. 160.

SATURDAY

BREAKFAST

   1 cup tomato juice
   1-egg (or egg substitute) omelet
   ½ cup grits
   1 teaspoon margarine
   5 slices melba toast
   1 cup skim milk
   Coffee or tea

LUNCH

   Sandwich: 1 ounce turkey, 1 ounce mozzarella on 1 toasted
      English muffin; 1 teaspoon mayonnaise; lettuce
   ½ cup vegetable juice
   ½ cantaloupe
   Noncaloric beverage

DINNER

   Veal Parmesan: 2 ounces veal, dipped in 1½ tablespoons
      bread crumbs and sautéed in nonstick pan in 2 teaspoons
      corn oil; 1 ounce mozzarella cheese; ½ cup Creole Sauce*
   ¾ cup boiled noodles
   Tossed salad: sliced tomatoes, onion, spinach, mushrooms,
      lettuce with vinegar dressing
   1 fresh pear
   Noncaloric beverage

SNACKS

   1 cup skim-milk orange junket
   5 vanilla wafers

   * See recipes starting on p. 160.

SAMPLE MENUS—1,800-CALORIE DIET

SUNDAY
BREAKFAST
½ cup orange juice
2 eggs (or egg substitute)
1 slice whole-wheat bread, toasted, with 1 teaspoon margarine
¾ cup corn flakes
½ banana
1 cup skim milk
Coffee or tea

LUNCH
3 ounces broiled steak
½ cup steamed broccoli with lemon wedge
Lettuce and tomato salad with 1 teaspoon salad dressing
Baked potato with 1 tablespoon sour cream
¼ honeydew melon
Noncaloric beverage

DINNER
3 ounces baked fillet of sole
Baked medium potato with 1 tablespoon sour cream
½ cup spinach
Tossed salad: carrots, tomatoes, mushrooms, zucchini, celery, cucumber, with low-calorie dressing
1 corn muffin
1 cup orange and grapefruit sections
Noncaloric beverage

SNACKS
1 cup skim milk
3 animal crackers

MONDAY
BREAKFAST
1 cup tomato juice
2 slices mozzarella cheese on 1 toasted English muffin with 1 strip crisp bacon

1 cup skim milk
Coffee or tea

LUNCH

Salad plate: ¾ cup crab meat, 2 teaspoons salad dressing,
3 tomatoes, cucumber slices, fresh asparagus on lettuce
with Spicy Vinegar Dressing*
½ cup cantaloupe
Iced tea with lemon and artificial sweetener or noncaloric
beverage

DINNER

3 ounces broiled barbecued chicken breast with low-calorie
Barbecue Sauce*
½ cup brown rice with ½ teaspoon margarine
½ cup green beans with ½ teaspoon margarine
Salad: ½ cup grated carrots with 2 tablespoons raisins and 2
teaspoons salad dressing on lettuce leaf
½ cup unsweetened applesauce with cinnamon
2 graham crackers
Noncaloric beverage

SNACKS

1 cup skim milk
¾ cup corn flakes

TUESDAY

BREAKFAST

1 cup orange and grapefruit sections
1 poached egg (or egg substitute)
1 ounce Canadian Bacon, grilled
1 toasted bagel with 1 tablespoon cream cheese
1 cup skim milk
Coffee or tea

* See recipes starting on p. 160.

LUNCH

3-ounce broiled hamburger on toasted hamburger roll; mustard

Dill pickle

1 cup coleslaw with 2 teaspoons low-calorie salad dressing on lettuce

1 medium apple

Noncaloric beverage

DINNER

3-ounce broiled lamb chop

½ cup parsleyed potatoes with 1 teaspoon margarine

½ cup yellow squash with ½ teaspoon margarine

½ cup red beet salad on lettuce with bermuda onion, oregano and low-calorie Spicy Vinegar Dressing*

1 small pita loaf

Low-calorie Lime Gelatin*

2 halves water-packed canned pears

Noncaloric beverage

SNACKS

1 cup skim-milk lemon junket

3 ginger snaps

WEDNESDAY

BREAKFAST

½ cup grapefruit juice

½ cup cottage cheese with cinnamon and nutmeg

2 slices toasted raisin bread with 1 teaspoon margarine

½ cup applesauce

1 cup skim milk

Coffee or tea

LUNCH

3 ounces sliced turkey on 2 slices rye bread; 1 teaspoon mayonnaise

½ cup tomato juice

Tossed salad with low-calorie dressing

* See recipes starting on p. 160.

1 three-inch wedge watermelon
Noncaloric beverage

DINNER

3 ounces grilled or broiled beef and chicken brochette (marinated in soy sauce) with ½ cup cherry tomatoes, small onion, green pepper, 2 pineapple slices
1 ear corn on the cob with 1 teaspoon margarine
½ cup steamed broccoli with 1 teaspoon margarine
1 slice French bread
½ cup blackberries
Noncaloric beverage

SNACKS

1 cup skim-milk plain yogurt
1 cup fresh strawberries

THURSDAY

BREAKFAST

⅔ cup pineapple juice
2-egg (or egg substitute) omelet
10 slices rye melba toast
1 teaspoon margarine
1 cup skim milk
Coffee or tea

LUNCH

Salad plate: ¾ cup low-fat cottage cheese, 6 grapes, 5 cherries, ½ fresh pear, ½ fresh peach
2 sesame bread sticks
1 cup vegetable juice
Noncaloric beverage

DINNER

3 ounces baked ham with parsley sprig
1 small baked sweet potato with 1 teaspoon margarine
½ cup fresh asparagus with 1 teaspoon margarine
Tossed salad with low-calorie dressing
1 slice rye bread
1 medium baked apple
Noncaloric beverage

SNACKS

1 cup chocolate skim milk
5 vanilla wafers

FRIDAY

BREAKFAST

¼ honeydew melon with lemon wedge
2 slices provolone cheese on 2 slices whole-wheat bread, grilled, with 1 teaspoon margarine
1 cup skim milk
Coffee or tea

LUNCH

3 ounces lean corned beef on 2 slices rye bread, mustard, horseradish, kosher pickle; lettuce and tomato
½ cup coleslaw with 1 teaspoon salad dressing
20 Bing cherries
Noncaloric beverage

DINNER

2-ounce veal cutlet, dipped in ½ tablespoon bread crumbs and cooked in 2 teaspoons oil
1 slice mozzarella cheese
½ cup Creole Sauce*
¾ cup steamed rice
½ cup green peas with small onions
Spinach salad with low-calorie dressing
1 slice Italian bread
24 grapes
Noncaloric beverage

SNACKS

1 cup skim milk
2 graham crackers

* See recipes starting on p. 160.

SATURDAY

BREAKFAST

½ cup orange juice
1 scrambled egg
1 slice baked ham
1 slice whole-wheat toast with 1 teaspoon margarine
⅓ cup bran cereal
½ banana
1 cup skim milk
Coffee or tea

LUNCH

Salad plate: ¾ cup water-packed tuna on lettuce with 2 teaspoons salad dressing
Relish plate: carrots, celery, radishes, cherry tomatoes
5 slices melba toast
1 cup blueberries
2 graham crackers
Noncaloric beverage

DINNER

3 ounces broiled haddock with lemon wedge
½ cup succotash with 1 teaspoon margarine
½ cup Brussels sprouts
Lettuce and tomato salad with low-calorie dressing
1 corn muffin
¼ honeydew with lemon slice
Noncaloric beverage

SNACKS

1 cup skim-milk plain yogurt
8 wheat thins

The following are recipes for the indicated foods in the sample
menus. They have been developed by the Johns Hopkins Hospital
Nutrition Department especially for weight-loss diets.

Low-Calorie Spicy Tomato Dressing

½ cup vinegar
½ cup tomato paste
Artificial sweetening equal to 5 teaspoons sugar
Black pepper
2 tablespoons lemon juice
Salt to taste

Mix all ingredients and pour over salad.

Makes about 1 cup.

Low-Calorie Spicy Vinegar Dressing

1 cup vinegar
2 tablespoons finely chopped onions
2 tablespoons onion juice
2 tablespoons lemon juice
Artificial sweetening equal to 6 teaspoons sugar
1 tablespoon dry mustard
1 teaspoon paprika
Dash of red pepper
Salt to taste

Mix all ingredients and pour over salad.

Makes about 1½ cups.

Spicy Salad Dressing

½ cup wine vinegar
½ teaspoon salt
½ clove garlic
1 tablespoon chopped parsley, oregano, or curry
Artificial sweetener to equal 1 teaspoon sugar

Mix all ingredients, and pour over salad.

Makes about 1½ cups.

Creole Sauce

1 onion, chopped
1 small green pepper, chopped
1 cup chopped celery
2 tomatoes, chopped, or 1 cup canned

Cook together with desired seasonings for 10 to 20 minutes. ½ cup equals one vegetable exchange.

Makes about 2½ cups.

Barbecue Sauce

Artificial sweetening equal to 1 teaspoon sugar
3 tablespoons cider vinegar
1 tablespoon grated onion
1½ teaspoons finely minced garlic
3 tablespoons Worcestershire sauce
¾ teaspoon salt
½ cup water
¼ cup tomato paste
¼ teaspoon paprika
½ teaspoon chili powder
3 drops Tabasco sauce
1 tablespoon prepared mustard

1. Mix ingredients in a quart saucepan.

2. Cook and stir until mixture boils. Lower heat, and cook 5 minutes longer.

Makes about 2 cups.

Cranberry Sauce

1 cup cranberries
¼ cup water
Artificial sweetening to taste (approximately equal to 12 teaspoons sugar)

1. Wash cranberries. Place them with water in a deep saucepan.

2. Cover, and cook until skins burst (about 10 minutes). Skim off the foam which collects on the top.

3. Add sweetening agent when slightly cool.

Makes about ½ cup sauce.

Lemon or Lime Gelatin

1 teaspoon unflavored gelatin
6 tablespoons water
2 tablespoons lemon or lime juice
Artificial sweetening to taste (approximately equal to 3 teaspoons sugar)
Fruit (optional)

1. Dissolve gelatin in cold water.

2. Bring lemon or lime juice to boil. Add to softened gelatin, and heat to the boiling point to dissolve the gelatin.

3. Add artificial sweetening.

4. Pour into mold, and chill. Part of the fruit allowed in the diet may be added if desired.

Makes one serving.

Coffee Almond Whip

1 teaspoon unflavored gelatin
2 tablespoons cold water
½ cup hot coffee
Artificial sweetening to taste (approximately equal to 3 teaspoons sugar)
⅛ teaspoon nutmeg
¼ teaspoon almond extract

1. Sprinkle gelatin over cold water. Let stand for 5 minutes. Add hot coffee, and stir until dissolved.

2. Add remaining ingredients. Chill until mixture begins to set.

3. Beat until fluffy with a rotary beater. Chill until firm.

Makes one serving.

Baked Custard

Artificial sweetening approximately equal to 1 teaspoon sugar
½ cup skim milk
1 egg, beaten
⅛ teaspoon salt

¼ teaspoon vanilla
Nutmeg

1. Dissolve artificial sweetening in a small amount of water, and combine with all remaining ingredients except the nutmeg.

2. Pour into large custard cup. Sprinkle with the nutmeg.

3. Place in shallow pan of hot water, and bake in moderate oven (350° F) about 50 minutes, or until knife inserted near edge of custard comes out clean.

Makes one serving.

12. Staying on the Diet Long Enough to Get Thin

I don't go on binges like you hear about. I don't eat whole cakes or a dozen doughnuts or anything like that. But I'm still a foodaholic, and what I do is eat perfectly normal meals but too much of them. If I'm feeling frustrated—and it usually has something to do with my job and the lack of appreciation I get there—I'll go out to lunch and eat enough for three people. Or I'll sit down to dinner, my wife puts a bowl of mashed potatoes on the table and, if she doesn't take it away, I'll finish all of it. Most of the time I don't do that, but often enough I essentially eat my frustrations.

—Marketing analyst, age 55

The first few days or weeks of a diet, for most of us, is an experience that arouses feelings of virtue, righteousness and great expectations. But then comes the most crucial and the hardest part, staying on the diet plan long enough to succeed at getting thin. At our clinic at Johns Hopkins we have amassed a vast collection of guidelines, helpful hints and useful information which have helped our patients become some of the most successful "losers" in the country.

You, too, can use these techniques, picking and choosing among them for those that make the diet plan work best for you. Only you can decide when and where to apply them, now that you know what kind of overeater you are.

You will discover some facts nobody ever told you that are additional weapons in your fight against fat. For example, did you know there are certain warning signs that will alert you to the imminent danger of diet disaster? Perhaps, too, you have never understood how your own internal body clock affects your eating habits and how you can use it now. Did you know that the third week of any diet is Quitter's Week, the time when the temptation to give up the latest battle is the strongest? You will find out how to deal with plateaus, which every serious dieter encounters, as well as the inevitable "cheating" episodes and the people who try to tempt you off your diet.

You will learn to persist until you are the shape you want to be. Don't fool yourself into thinking that a permanent weight loss can result from a temporary effort. Dieting is hard work, and you must expect occasional setbacks. Most overweight people, especially the devotees of the light-bulb philosophy of dieting (on again, off again), make a deal with themselves. "OK," they'll say, "I'll suffer until May, and I'll lose forty pounds." Then, they figure, that's it. Done. Finished. Thin. Forget it. Resume former life.

But it doesn't work that way. When they resume their former life-styles, the ones that made them overweight in the first place, they are soon right back where they started from—fat. That's why it's important to continue applying what you learn here to your eating behavior.

THE CARDINAL RULES

1. **Be patient.** Overweight people are not famous for their patience. They want to be thin right *now*, or maybe in two weeks. They want to be visibly thinner every morning. But to get off the diet merry-go-round, time is essential. You didn't become overweight overnight, so you can't expect to undo the damage overnight either. Be prepared for a consistent and steady weight loss because an overly rapid loss only brings a quick rebound. On the University Medical Diet, you will lose perhaps two or three pounds (or more) the first week, then a pound or two a week after that. You will not feel unduly deprived, you will be eating healthily and you will have time to observe and change the ways you have been using food to your disadvantage.

2. **Don't set unrealistic goals** for how many pounds you will lose. Don't insist to yourself, for example, "I'm going to lose sixty pounds in four months," or "I'll be size twelve by July" if you are size eighteen in May. Just decide how much you are going to shed this week—and do it.

3. **Live from meal to meal.** Make it from breakfast through those few hours until lunch. Then simply concentrate on

getting safely through until dinner. Breaking your time into small components makes it easier to resist temptation.

4. **Remember you have the option to be thinner.** Every time you put the wrong foods in your mouth, you are opting to be fat. Do you want to be thin, or would you rather have that chocolate cake?

5. **Beware of Quitter's Week.** The third week of any diet is usually the most dangerous. By this time the novelty has worn off, and the new regimen has become routine. You are tired of watching what you eat. And most important, you have rid yourself of the water that causes rapid weight loss at the beginning of any consistent cut in calories. Now you are working on your fat, which takes longer to go. Your resolve may weaken, and you must be especially careful not to become a diet casualty.

6. **Plot your plateaus.** Weight loss is never consistent, never the same every week. Like all dieters, you will reach plateaus, periods when your weight won't budge downward despite your best efforts. These plateaus are normal, and they will pass.

Plateaus begin most often, our studies show, between the seventh and eighth weeks and the third and fourth months, and neither men nor women are immune to them. They tend to occur about every four months and usually last about two weeks, though for some people they may continue for as long as a month or two.

The heavier you are, the more plateaus you are likely to encounter because as you rid yourself of a significant amount of fat and you get smaller, you require fewer calories to maintain your body.

Caution! Warning! Remember that everyone loses weight in an erratic pattern. This is normal. Don't blow your plans now. You will start losing again. Read on for ways we have discovered to cope with plateaus.

7. **Forgive yourself.** When you stray from the straight and narrow and go on a binge, forget it. Don't waste time on

guilt. Nobody's perfect. Simply go right back on the program immediately. Don't wait until tomorrow or next Monday. If you do, it's like swiping a nickel and deciding you might as well rob the bank. The consequences are very different.

8. **Anticipate.** You are certain to hit emotional rough spots, so be ready for them. Accept the fact that certain situations, people, happenings cause anxiety and the desire to eat. It's much better to face your emotions and deal with them than to believe a dish of ice cream will make them go away.

9. **Never skip meals.** This is the most destructive habit most overweight people have. They think that by skipping breakfast or lunch or both, they are speeding up their weight loss. But almost invariably they make up for it later, eating too much because they become ravenous or wasting their caloric allotment on nonnutritious food. You will end up fatigued, enervated and discouraged.

10. **Prepare for the "down" times.** Feeling out of sorts, irritable, tired, depressed sometimes accompanies the first couple of weeks on a new diet program, though some people sail through the initial weeks feeling euphoric and enthusiastic and *then* crash. Your body needs time to adjust to lower calories. Don't use the down times as an excuse to quit.

11. **Don't be a diet bore.** If you become totally involved with what you are eating and which way the scale is moving, it's no fun and certainly is a bore for everyone around you.

12. **Don't be obsessed by the scales.** Your weight constantly fluctuates because of your daily body rhythms, your hormonal output, your water retention and the actual contents of your bladder and digestive tract, which can hold many pounds of food. Your weight may vary a couple of pounds in a single day. Try to resist jumping onto the scales every hour or even every day. Weigh yourself, undressed, once a week at the same time of day.

13. **Review the evidence.** Whenever you feel an inappropriate urge to eat, review the reasons you overeat and examine your moods. Reread the first few chapters of this book. If you don't understand the problem, you are going to eat when you're under the influence. If necessary, begin keeping the Food Diary again as a way to monitor yourself.

14. **Smarten up.** Start paying more attention to your appearance. Get a new hairstyle; give yourself a manicure; alter your clothes to fit; sew on buttons; take pride in yourself. You are on your way to a new shape, and you may as well look good doing it.

15. **Take charge of yourself.** Ask yourself, when you look in a mirror, "Is anyone forcing me to look like that? Do I have to put up with that body? Do I have the power to change it?" Then acknowledge that *you* are the responsible party. Your body is the result of what *you* have been doing with what nature gave you. Unless you take responsibility, all the books and diets in the world won't help you.

Weight-Loss Gimmicks to Avoid

In a survey made at our clinic, we found that 74 percent of the overweight population is willing to "try anything once" to lose weight. But many highly publicized weight-loss methods are dangerous, and others are useless:

• Appetite suppressants are *never* recommended. They can be hazardous and at best are ineffective. Diet pills are among the most widely sold drugs in the United States. In 1981 about 4 million Americans took more than 10 billion doses of products containing a drug called PPA (phenylpropanolamine), the active ingredient in most appetite suppressants and the one accused of causing the most severe side effects especially for people with certain medical conditions. Other active ingredients in some diet drugs are diuretics, which give a false impression of weight loss (because they cause water loss, not fat loss); benzocaine, an anesthetic that numbs the taste buds; a thyroid extract which boosts metabolic rate; digitalis to increase heart rate. Caffeine is often added as a stimulant.

Though some appetite suppressants speed up weight loss, they lose their effectiveness within a few weeks, and cause a rapid regain of weight in a rebound effect.

• Body wraps for spot reducing are ineffective and may also be dangerous. Cloths soaked in a chemical solution and wrapped around parts of the body, they induce excessive perspiration, compression of tissue and temporary dehydration.

• Rubber or plastic reducing suits, stockings, chin and neck trimmers, heated abdomen belts don't work. Besides, they may cut off circulation and cause debilitating dehydration. They will only make you *seem* thinner for a few hours until the water you have lost reappears.

• Vibrating machines promise weight reduction with no effort. They are ineffective.

• Massage feels marvelous, and it can take the kinks out of your muscles; but it won't get rid of fat. Besides, it may injure the skin and subcutaneous connective tissue and cause broken capillaries.

• Antacids used to depress appetite can raise blood pressure because of their sodium content and can mask symptoms of gastrointestinal disorders.

• Hot tubs, steam baths and saunas do not produce weight loss. They merely cause a temporary loss of water.

• Starch blockers, a recent diet fad, are under investigation by the Food and Drug Administration because of reported illnesses and side effects associated with the tablets. These pills, made from raw bean protein, are claimed to block the digestion of starch in the intestines so you can eat all you want without absorbing it. Aside from being potentially dangerous for some people, such as diabetics, these drugs have not been proved to work, and the possible long-term effects, particularly resulting from a deficiency of nutrients available only from carbohydrates, may make them risky for your health. Serious side effects include diarrhea, intestinal cramps and possible aggravation of blood-clotting disorders.

HOW TO HANDLE A PLATEAU

Aside from enduring it, there are some effective ways we recommend to give yourself a slight push off a plateau:

Drink water. Water often acts as a catalyst. Have a glassful ten minutes before every meal (it also takes the edge off your appetite) and more during it.

Review your diet. If necessary, start keeping your Food Diary again. You may discover that little dibs and dabs of extra nourishment have been slipping between your lips, unnoticed. But a few dibs and dabs can add up to a lot of calories. Be honest with yourself. Maybe this isn't a plateau, but a minor breakdown.

If, on review, you find you are pristine and pure, then you will know you are experiencing a perfectly normal physiological adjustment to the changes you have made in your eating and activity patterns. Don't panic. It will end.

Increase your physical activity. Exercise may be the most important and effective step you can take, especially if you are certain you are eating the prescribed number of calories. It may be the only way you can continue to lose enough weight to keep your spirits up. Done vigorously enough, it can promptly raise your metabolism so that less fat is put into storage.

Reduce your calories slightly, but never go below 1,000 a day without your doctor's supervision. If your smaller body now requires fewer calories than you have been eating, you will soon find out. And you are giving yourself a physiological as well as psychological shot in the arm, perhaps sufficient to get you going again. You may wish to go back to the Starter Diet for a week or two.

You can cut calories by eating smaller portions of meat and eating low-calorie fish. Try using less salt on your food. Choose foods lower in calories but more filling.

If the scale doesn't show any change, try a tape measure. Very often, with increased exercise, your fat tissue is burned off and your muscle mass increases. Though your weight remains the same, you are getting thinner because a pound of muscle has much less volume than a pound of fat. You may be losing inches that don't show up on the scale.

Facts About Water

• The best diuretic is *water.* It acts as a catalyst for the body to decrease its water retention. Drink six to eight glasses a day. Do not take a chemical diuretic to help you lose weight. It may be harmful, and it is certainly ineffective because the water will return to the tissues as soon as you stop taking it. Diuretics should be used only when prescribed by a physician for a specific physical condition that requires water loss. Water not only is the best and most effective diuretic but is also cheap, safe, and healthy.

• Most of the weight loss during the first couple of weeks on a low-calorie diet is *water.* That is true for *any* diet, but especially a high-protein regimen. Don't get overexcited by the descending numbers on the scale.

• Overweight people are much more likely than others to sprinkle salt indiscriminately over their food. They also use condiments—many of them salt-laden—more freely. Salt promotes water retention. If you want to diminish retention, cut back on the sprinkling. The average diet includes up to 200 times as much salt as the body requires.

• Some diet sodas contain large amounts of sodium (salt). If you drink many a day, you may find you are retaining excess water. Drink water instead. Remember, too, there is a high salt content in many prepared foods, such as some canned soups and vegetables, preserved delicatessen meats, dried fruits, pickles, TV dinners, etc.

• Many women easily gain several pounds just before their menstrual periods because of increased water retention. If this happens to you, don't confuse it with a true weight gain, which consists of fat tissue.

HOW TO HANDLE CHEATING

There is no perfect dieter. In all our experience in the last fifteen years at our weight-loss clinic, we have yet to see one. It is normal to detour from the direct route to thinness occasionally, eating more than you should, especially during periods of stress or excitement. Most dieters are always restraining themselves from overeating, consciously consuming less than they really desire, so it's entirely understandable that they'll break out now and then like a prisoner who comes upon an unlocked gate.

But though cheating is normal and inevitable, it must be kept to a minimum, or you have defeated your own purpose. Be honest with yourself. Nobody may see you gobbling that chocolate bar or taking yet another portion of mashed potatoes swimming in butter, but you're still not getting away with it. The calories will add up to fat, and the fat will show up on the scale. If you have decided you truly want to lose weight, learn to keep your cheating under control or all your other efforts will be canceled out.

Confess!

The technique we have found works best for almost everyone who's making an all-out effort to be thin is to confess your dietary sins—not to your priest or a doctor or your mother but to yourself. Keep a Cheat Sheet. This is a miniversion of the Food Diary that every new member of our groups records for two weeks.

In your purse or shirt pocket, place a small notebook and a pencil, ready for action. Every time you eat even a bite or a sip of food that is out of bounds, not on your diet plan—and we mean even a few peanuts, three teaspoons of ice cream, anything—write it down. This impresses the happening on your mind so it won't slip by without notice.

Also note the date, the time, the place, the company, your emotional state. At the end of each week try to approximate the number of calories you have added to your basic diet, and decide if they have influenced your weight. One of our patients, a middle-aged man, reviewed his Cheat Sheets for four weeks and came to the conclusion that his extra nibbling had cost him four pounds. Consider this: A snack or a drink worth only 100 calories each per day adds up to 36,500 calories a year. That's ten extra pounds you don't need.

Analyze the circumstances under which you cheated so you'll be able to anticipate future episodes and ward them off before they happen.

After a while, by its mere presence in your pocket and your mind, the Cheat Sheet will serve as an excellent conditioner. You'll find you don't want to write anything down in your little notebook, so you won't stray so often. At the least you will stop and think before going ahead. When you realize you'll have to report that chocolate chip cookie you are about to eat, maybe you will decide not to eat it after all.

All Calories Count

Remember, all calories going down your throat count, whether or not you note them down. So thinking it doesn't matter because nobody knows and you haven't recorded it means only that you have tricked yourself. If you can't play fair with yourself, you have set yourself up for another diet another day.

BEWARE: SABOTEURS AT WORK

Nobody who's decided to lose weight fails to run into diet saboteurs, people who try—usually unconsciously—to tempt you to eat what you shouldn't. The saboteurs are often the people closest to you—your spouse, your mother, your friends—who for their own reasons cannot bear the idea that you are getting thinner or truly think you are in no need of change. They worry about you, fear losing you or their hold over you, hate to see you deprived of one of life's pleasures, are afraid you are wasting away, view you as a threat or mourn the loss of your company as a fellow eater.

Whatever their reasons and whatever their motives, you must learn how to cope with diet saboteurs because if you don't, you will never be thin.

The Sabotaging Spouse

Probably most common among the tempters are the spouses of those who are trying to slim down. In fact, we have found that in 35 percent of over 4,000 cases of true obesity which we studied, the husbands or wives made an earnest effort to keep their mates fat.

Why? Often a husband (or, less frequently, a wife) who lacks self-esteem and self-confidence feels threatened by a wife (or husband) who is becoming more attractive and perhaps independent of him, no longer needing an "inferior" mate.

Sometimes a wife feels her delectable cooking is her major contribution to the marriage and wants to hold onto that source of praise. Perhaps a husband thinks he, too, must go on a diet and shape up if his wife does, or a wife fears she'll have to give up desserts and snacks and never have a tasty tidbit in the house. Often a couple's chief form of entertainment has been good food, new restaurants and experimental calorie-rich cooking, and one spouse's new plans spoil the fun.

Couples with poor sexual relationships can blame them on the fat wife or the overweight husband, but without the fat, rationalization for failure is gone. Or perhaps extramarital straying, based on the unappealing shape of a mate (or at least excused by it), is threatened by the emerging slimness, eliciting offerings of forbidden foods and favorite dishes. Sometimes the man is sexually attracted to overweight women or the woman to fat men. Our study showed that the majority of men who prefer heavy women had fat mothers or their first satisfactory sexual experiences with large women.

"Go On, Have a Little Piece"

Not only husbands and wives but other family members are frequently the unwitting saboteurs of a weight-loss plan. How often have you heard, "But I made this especially for you! You've always loved spaghetti." Or, "You're getting too thin; you look drawn. Take a little more pudding."

Mothers, of course, are noted food pushers since their role traditionally has been that of the nurturers of the family. They may consider their meals symbols of their love and concern and offer them as expressions of giving. Nevertheless, they can keep you overweight.

Other relatives and friends—usually women—who love to cook and entertain take your refusal of their offerings as rejections of them. You may be taking away one of their greatest pleasures: your enjoyment of their talents in the kitchen and their generosity as hosts.

Sometimes there is genuine concern for your health, especially in ethnic or family groups in which plumpness has always been equated with well-being. For some people, visible bone structure symbolizes deprivation. And if you are actually losing too much weight, becoming too thin for your frame, they may be right!

"It's a Special Occasion. It Won't Hurt You to Have It Just This Once"

Are you a new threat to friends or colleagues for dates, jobs, admiration, power? As you become more socially acceptable and attractive to yourself as well as others, you may find your relationships are undergoing a distinct change. Sometimes other people who feel threatened by you are overweight themselves and want company. Or thin, they need to feel superior. Maybe they miss you as an eating companion, someone who was always good for a hot fudge sundae or a quick trip to the deli, or as an always available baby-sitter, listener, worker, laugher, grateful for their time and attention. Let's face it, you are more comfortable for them *fat*.

How to Hang In Despite Them

Whatever the reasons your family and friends and acquaintances have for luring you to foods you shouldn't eat or second helpings when you've had enough, hold your ground. Don't get angry, pathetic, petulant, hostile. Simply state your case, which is that you are determined this time to lose weight, you are following the diet plan of the Health, Weight and Stress Program at Johns Hopkins, and you don't care for any, thank you. Tell them you appreciate their concern and you love their cooking, but it is very important to you to be thinner. If that fails, simply say firmly, "Thank you, I'm sure it's delicious, but I don't care for any right now." Above all, don't whine, "Gee, I'd really love it, but I can't have it. You see, I'm on this diet. . . ." They will be tempted to coax.

In our classes we recommend that you arrange to discuss the situation openly and empathetically with the other person, if that person is close to you, in an effort to explain yourself and ask for help instead of hindrance. Diet saboteurs will usually recognize when they are making surreptitious efforts to torpedo your diet plans or that you interpret their interest in your health as damaging to your resolve. Talk it over, exchange your views and do both of you a favor.

Early Warning Signals:
Indications You May Be About to Go Off Your Diet

From our thousands of patients we have gleaned a short list of flashing yellow lights, warning signals of impending abandonment of all best-laid plans to lose weight.

When you spot any of these signs, watch out. Start using some of the techniques that have helped you. Don't let inertia and an urge to let nature take its course ("I told you, I have no will power") block your intentions to improve your body.

1. You compare yourself to other people who are losing more weight on the same calories or people who don't have to watch their calories. You feel envious or angry and terribly deprived.

2. You are spending an unusual amount of time watching television.

3. You have cravings for specific foods.

4. You start skipping breakfast (or lunch) again.

5. Strolling past a bakery or a delicatessen, you decide to go in and buy some treats for the family. You're not going to eat any, of course.

6. You start blaming your husband, your mother-in-law, your cat, your boss or your children for annoying and upsetting you so much that you are getting urges to eat foods you know you shouldn't.

7. You notice you are watching other people eat.

8. You're discouraged because you hardly lost any weight this week despite adherence to your diet plan.

9. People are beginning to notice your weight loss and to say, "You are looking marvelous. You're losing weight, aren't you?" This is the moment when many people, especially women, allow their fear of thinness to overwhelm their desire to become what they have always said they wanted to be—thin.

10. You start to cheat a little here and there, thinking, "What does it matter, this tiny piece of cake?" Or you increase your portions. And you don't write it down.

ANTISTRESS TACTICS

If you are a typical overeater, stress sends you directly to the kitchen, the doughnut shop or the vending machine in search of a bite to eat. We have found in our classes that with only a few practice sessions, every stress eater can learn to become more relaxed. When you are freer of tension, your blood will flow more readily through expanded blood vessels, your heart and respiration rate will decrease, your digestive tract will work more efficiently, you can identify and deal with your problems better—and you can stop automatically turning to food in an effort to set things right.

Try these relaxation techniques, and see if they don't help you stay on your diet. Repeat as needed the ones that help you most.

1. **Take a bath.** An ordinary bath, neither too hot nor too cold, but warm, just a few degrees above body temperature. Soak for at least fifteen minutes.

2. **Slow down.** Have a sit-down breakfast, giving yourself sufficient time to enjoy it without feeling rushed. That means, obviously, you must get up a little earlier than you have been. Don't procrastinate and then rush off to work or an appointment in a panic. Take a real lunch break; that means you don't eat at your desk with a pencil in your hand or standing up in front of the refrigerator. Plan your food, sit down and eat it slowly. Take a walk during your lunch hour. In the evening rest or exercise before having dinner. Hurrying produces stress.

3. **Untense your muscles.** Sit in a comfortable chair or lie down on your bed. Tighten all the muscles in your face. Frown. Press your lips together. Squeeze your eyes shut.

Tense your body; clench your fists; draw your shoulders up around your ears. Stiffen your buttocks and your abdomen; brace your legs. Hold the physical tension while you count slowly to twenty.

Then let it all go! Feel the tension flow out of your body. Beginning at your feet and progressing to the top of your head, relax all your muscles one by one. Let your toes droop, your legs relax, your stomach sag, your shoulders fall. Make your jaw go slack; relax your mouth; release your cheeks, all the little muscles around your eyes, eyelids and forehead, even the top of your scalp. Let your hands hang down at your sides, and feel the tension run out of your fingertips, making them feel tingly and heavy. Maintain the relaxation for five minutes.

4. **Visualize.** Sit or lie down in a comfortable, quiet place where you won't be disturbed. Take a deep breath through your nose, and let it out through your mouth. Slowly. Three or four times.

Now relax your muscles, one by one, from your feet to your head, until you feel like limp spaghetti. Turn off your mind. For five minutes visualize a beautiful, serene place where you are all alone, perhaps stretched out on a beautiful, warm, sandy beach. Feel the warm, silky sand on your back and the gentle rays of the sun on your face. Picture wisps of soft clouds floating across the blue sky like gray chiffon, and feel the gentle breeze wafting across your supine body, the sun making little diamonds on the waves as the sea laps gently at the nearby shore. Your eyes are softly closed, and your cheekbones feel tight in the sun.

As you lie there, the tiredness and tension run right out of your body into the sand, and you feel slimmer and lighter and happier. You feel relaxed and at peace.

Now take a deep breath in. Let it out. Count backward from ten to one, slowly and rhythmically. Open your eyes and stretch.

5. **Talk to yourself.** Just before you go to sleep every night, give yourself a pep talk. Say to yourself, "Tomorrow I am going to stick to my diet plan and get my exercise. I will be thinner. I will think thin. I will eat thin."

In the morning, just before you get out of bed, think of yourself as you want to look when you have lost your projected weight. Visualize your body, your clothes, your energy. Repeat your vows.

If it helps, and it often does with our members, talk to yourself on a tape that you can play back morning and night and any other time you need help. Speak in soft, serene, unhurried tones, because this is really a form of self-hypnosis. Or have someone else make the tape for you. We have found that a male voice, if you are a woman, and a female voice, if you are a man, are the most effective.

You may also want to make a relaxation tape, putting into words the visualizations described in tip number 4.

6. **Meditate.** Learn meditation, an ancient technique that actually lowers blood pressure, oxygen consumption and heart rate by blocking the effects of the hormones made by the body under stress. Meditation—or relaxation response—provides time out for your mind, giving respite and rest, and can help you calm down and handle your hassles with more perspective and serenity. We have found that because it reduces the inner tensions that come from living in today's stress-filled world, it also goes a long way toward helping you cope with your day and therefore your diet.

In simplified form, here is one way to meditate:

Sit in a comfortable position in an upright chair. Don't lie down or lean your head back, or you may go to sleep. Choose a place where you won't be disturbed. Lock your pets out. Tell your children you will be available again in twenty minutes. Turn off the telephone. Though perfect quiet is the best setting, it's not necessary. You can meditate on a train, in a hotel lobby, in your office with the door closed, anywhere out of range of individual voices, music or loud noises.

Close your eyes, and sit quietly for a minute or two. Consciously relax all your muscles, from head to toes.

Now start repeating silently to yourself a preselected meaningless sound—perhaps *om-m-m-m* or *ming-g-g-g* or any other sound you choose. Just remember this will continue to be your mantra, so pick a sound you can live with without changing. Repeat the sound for twenty minutes. (Open one eye, and peek at the clock. After a few weeks you will be able to sense when your twenty minutes have elapsed.)

Don't force yourself to say your sound. Just do it as effortlessly as possible. Your mind will wander off. When you realize it has, simply remind yourself of your mantra and resume; on the other hand, once you have realized you are daydreaming, don't continue to do so. Go back to the mantra. And don't be concerned if you don't say your sound too much of the time. The effects are cumulative, and after a few weeks you will feel the difference in yourself.

After twenty minutes stop saying the mantra, and sit quietly again for two minutes. Slowly open your eyes.

Meditate twice a day, before breakfast and before dinner.

Will More Frequent Bowel Movements Help in Weight Loss?

No, not permanently. They result only in the temporary loss of water plus the weight of the waste material. Forcing yourself to have bowel movements more often than normal (for some people, that is every day; for others, every two or three days) by eating too much fiber or taking laxatives is dangerous. It can result in the breakdown of muscle and organ tissue and the elimination of essential vitamins and minerals. A new fad diet, promoted in a best-selling book, is based on losing weight through diarrhea and has been denounced by reputable medical authorities everywhere.

It does, however, make sense to eat a diet that contains a reasonable amount of fiber foods. This helps shorten the length of time fats and sugars remain in the digestive tract, giving them less time to be absorbed by the intestines. In other words, fiber decreases the transit time and may increase your bowel movements or at least regularize them. But fiber must not be consumed in such amounts that your diet does not contain a balance of the nutrients a healthy body requires.

YOUR CIRCADIAN RHYTHMS CAN HELP YOU LOSE WEIGHT

Are you a morning person, a lark, who wakes up chirping, cheerful and energetic? Do you wind down as the day progresses and like to get to bed at a decent hour? Or are you an owl, a night person, who loves to sleep late, spends the early hours of the day half asleep, and comes to life only sometime during the afternoon? You may be neither a classic owl nor a lark, but you will certainly tend to be more one type than the other because of your personal biological rhythms.

Studies at Johns Hopkins have shown that our biological clocks—more scientifically known as circadian rhythms—have an important influence on what we eat and when we eat it. And some researchers have even claimed that food converts to fat more easily when it is consumed at one time of day than another.

Dr. Charles Ehret, senior researcher in The Division of Biological and Medical Research at the Argonne National Laboratory near Chicago, is an authority on circadian rhythms. He is the person who dubbed the day people larks and the night people owls. Using his terms, we will discuss the differences between them in terms of weight.

Overweight Owls

Overweight owls, we have discovered among the thousands of people who have gone through our program, are likely to be extroverts who thoroughly enjoy their food and eat plenty of it. They tend to skip breakfast, not only because they get up so late that they have little time for it but also because their lack of morning energy depresses their appetite. Anyway, they figure, they have thereby eliminated a few calories. But they make up for it, double time, later in the day, especially at night, when they are their most sociable.

Owls are usually flexible sorts who don't easily adhere to fixed schedules. Their eating patterns reflect this, making them erratic in the times they eat, as well as in the amounts and varieties of what they consume. They often specialize in high-calorie binges, followed by remorseful dieting.

Overweight Larks

Overweight larks, on the other hand, live more structured lives as a rule. They tend to be introspective and controlled and plan their food much more carefully than owls, who usually eat whatever is available at the moment. They are early risers who eat breakfast, lunch and dinner, usually well balanced. Their trouble is that they also eat *in between* breakfast, lunch and dinner—and before they go to bed as well. But when they are dieting, they stay with it better than owls.

What Makes Them Different?

Owls and larks differ because their body clocks operate on different schedules. Each person's life proceeds in a predictable pattern of circadian cycles that occur roughly every twenty-four hours (not to be confused with the so-called biorhythms, which are essentially folklore). These physiological pacemakers affect every system and activity in our bodies, from heartbeat (which can vary in the same individual up to thirty beats per minute at different times of day), to blood pressure (usually higher late in the day), temperature (which may change as much as two degrees daily), production of hormones and other body chemicals circulating throughout the bloodstream to energy levels, memory, physical ability, mathematical acuity, even taste discrimination and appetite.

Different Timetables for Different People

Each of us has our own daily physiological set of cycles that literally make us different people at different times of day or night. The cycles repeat themselves around every twenty-four hours, though they can be thrown out of sync temporarily by such disturbances as lack of sleep, jet travel, illness, changing work shifts, caffeine consumption and changes in mealtimes.

While owls may lag an hour or more behind the larks, for most of us, body temperature is its lowest in the early hours of the morning and highest around six in the evening. About half of our adrenal hormones are secreted into the bloodstream before we wake up in the morning, and early in the day there is a surge in the

production of corticotrophin, a pituitary hormone. In the morning, when these hormones are at their highest levels, our senses of
taste and smell are usually at a low ebb.

Heartbeat, respiration and physical ability usually peak
around midday, while blood pressure, ability to clot blood and
weight are generally highest by evening.

As body temperature and the other vital processes rise during
the day, most of us start feeling more energetic, and we are at our
best when our temperature is as its normal high point. At midday
or in the early afternoon the typical person is best prepared to
handle tasks requiring good memory, mathematical skills and eye-
hand coordination. Afternoons we tend to be physically stronger
and faster.

The body clock, among all its others influences, affects the way
we eat. For one thing, **the average person's senses of taste and
smell become sharper and more discriminating as the day goes
on,** so we are more likely to be adventurous in our choice of foods
at dinner than at breakfast. And our favorite goodies become more
and more appealing late in the day, especially for owls.

Moods and attitudes also have their corresponding high and
low points throughout the span of a day, affecting when and what
we eat. This is particularly true for psychological overeaters, who
respond to emotions with food. Low points for many people arrive
in late afternoon; for others, early mornings or evenings are when
they are most likely to feel depressed or anxious and so turn to
food.

An added feature: **The rhythm of metabolism may make food
more fattening at one time of day than another. Most of us convert food to energy most efficiently in the morning, while later in
the day it is more likely to be stored as fat.** This means that if our
bodies are particularly sensitive to this fluctuation, it makes more
sense to eat most of our calories at breakfast and lunch than at
night. Besides, a high-protein breakfast helps the brain produce
body chemicals that increase alertness and energy that last for
many hours.

Check Out Your Own Body Clock

If you get in touch with your daily pattern of peaks and valleys, both physical and emotional, you can use this information to

help control your weight. You will discover the times when food tempts you most, when your trouble spots are likely to appear, the moods that routinely recur, triggering automatic yearnings for food. Knowing your timetable can help you take advantage of your up times and guard against your downs.

Here's how to do it:

For at least a week and preferably two weeks, measure your physical, mental and emotional condition *at least every two hours* during your waking hours, starting *before* you get out of bed in the morning. Take your temperature; check your pulse; note your mood, energy level, task performance, appetite and the food you have eaten since the last notation.

Make a series of daily charts like this (or photocopy this one):

Date	Time	Temp.	Pulse	Mood	Energy Level	Task Performance	Appetite	Foo

Instructions

Temperature. Use an oral thermometer, and after shaking it down, place it under your tongue for three minutes. Record the reading, to one-tenth of a degree.

Pulse. You will need a watch or clock with a second hand. Place your thumb and first two fingers on either side of your throat just under your jawbone. Count the number of times your heart beats in one minute. This is your pulse rate.

Mood. Note whether you are feeling happy, contented, depressed, angry, excited, indifferent, bored, normal, apprehensive, relaxed, lonely, etc.

Energy Level. Jot down whether you are energetic, mentally alert, tired, somewhat tired, physically strong, etc.

Task Performance. Measure your perceived ability to accomplish tasks. Can you concentrate? Are your coordination and organizational ability good? Do you make mistakes, take too much time? Overall do you feel you are doing a good job?

Appetite. Choose strong, medium or low intensity.

Food. Write down what you have consumed in the past two hours.

From your daily records, you will quickly discern a pattern. Are you the happiest, most energetic, most able at a particular time? When does your brain seem to function best? Do you feel topnotch when your pulse and temperature are highest? Do you eat more at certain times? When does your desire for food seem to be most intense? Does it correlate with physical or emotional lows and highs?

Beware the Ninety-Minute Syndrome

Within the usual daily patterns of the body there is a shorter series of cycles of ups and downs, according to Dr. Ronald Gatty, who has made an intensive study of biological rhythms. About every ninety minutes throughout the day our ability to concentrate and focus tends to sag. We become restless, scattered, distractable. This is the time we especially want to put something into our mouths. Some people chew on pencils, bite their fingernails, fiddle with paper clips or pour another cup of coffee. We who tend to be overweight think of food.

But hold off. In about fifteen minutes your natural downswing will be curving upward again. If you can't get by with harmless pencil chewing, try a low-calorie snack or a big glass of water, sugarless gum, or, best of all possible choices, take an exercise break.

Take note of your best hours, when you can think clearly, plan your eating strategy and follow through. Keep an eye out for the times when danger lurks and it is easiest to give in to the temptation to overeat. Using the 112 Useful Tips and Tricks to Conquer Compulsive Eating listed in the next chapter, you can take evasive action that will distract you from the need to pave over your low moods with food. If you note that the times you especially want to eat compulsively arrive at certain hours of the day, you'll know you aren't really hungry but are simply experiencing your normal daily mood swings. Remember: This, too, shall pass. Once you know, for example, that you tend to feel depressed, fearful, anxious or simply fatigued at four in the afternoon, you can more easily fend off the food with distracting activities.

Special to Overweight Owls

Your most dangerous times, the hours you are most likely to abandon your diet and succumb to the temptation to eat too much of the wrong foods, are most likely to be between 8:30 and 10:00 P.M. Other precarious moments usually arrive in late afternoon and, if you are up and around, in the wee hours of the morning. Be particularly careful on Friday and Saturday nights because you tend to be a social eater.

Special to Overweight Larks

Your prime danger time for overeating is midmorning, around 10:30 A.M.; the next comes most often about four in the afternoon. Be sure to include protein in breakfast and lunch, and if you are going to a dinner party, preload yourself with a protein snack.

EATING OUT

Eating out can be just as much a feast when you are dieting as when you aren't. Making wise choices becomes a habit, and it is fun to pick and choose the best foods from a varied menu. Once you've adjusted to the exchange lists and have learned size of portions, you can enjoy gourmet meals at home or away from home.

Some Helpful Hints to Follow in a Restaurant

Foods to Select	Foods to Avoid

1. Appetizers

Foods to Select	Foods to Avoid
Broth, bouillon or consommé	Cream soups or chowders Breads and crackers (unless used as a bread choice)
Tomato juice, vegetable juice, unsweetened juice or fresh fruit	Sweetened juices or seafood cocktails (unless they are part of your meat choice)

2. Beverages

Foods to Select	Foods to Avoid
Coffee or tea (hot or iced) Skim milk (if in meal plan) Unsweetened juice (if used as a fruit choice) Tomato or vegetable juice (if used as a vegetable choice)	Coffee with added cream and sugar, dried creamers, chocolate milk, milk shakes, cocoa, sodas, sweetened juices, punch, sweetened sodas, presweetened lemonade, Kool-Aid or iced tea

3. Bread and Bread Substitutes

Foods to Select	Foods to Avoid
Baked or boiled potato	Potatoes: fried, mashed escalloped or creamed
Steamed rice, noodles, spaghetti, macaroni	Macaroni and cheese, spaghetti with sauce, creamed sauces
Corn on the cob, lima beans, succotash, green peas	Creamed vegetables
Hamburger roll, loaf bread, plain dinner roll, bread sticks, melba toast, pita bread (small loaf), hard roll, English muffin, bagel, saltines, tortilla or taco shell (all to be used in the specified amounts)	Bread dressings, biscuits, pancakes, sweet rolls, coffee cake, rum buns, crepes, doughnuts Baked beans, corn pudding, french fries

4. Desserts

Foods to Select	Foods to Avoid
Fresh fruit in season, ice cream (½ cup scoop equals 1 bread plus 2 fat choices) Fresh Fruit cup	Pudding, gelatin, cake, pie, pastry, cookies, ices, sherbets

Foods to Select	Foods to Avoid

5. Entrée

Broiled, baked, roasted or poached lean meat, fish or poultry

Eggs, poached, boiled, or plain omelets

Fatty or fried breaded meats, meats with gravies and sauces, barbecued meats, stews and casseroles

Egg salad, fried or scrambled eggs

6. Fats

Margarine, mayonnaise, salad dressing, sour cream, bacon (only as fat choices; then watch your portion sizes)

Fried foods, gravies, cream sauces, fat added during cooking

7. Relishes

Free vegetables, such as cucumbers, radishes, and lettuce (unless they are to be used as part of vegetable exchange)

Mustard, dill, sour or kosher pickles, horseradish

Sweet pickles, pickled beets, olives, mushrooms (unless used as a vegetable), pickle relish, pickled onions, pickled fruits

8. Salads

Tossed salads, lettuce heart, raw vegetables, carrots, celery, spinach, cottage cheese and fresh fruit (as part of meal if a fruit choice)

Ask that dressing not be added. Request vinegar and/or lemon wedge; or use French or Italian dressing or mayonnaise as a fat choice

Gelatin salads, salads with mayonnaise, whipped cream or toppings, coleslaw with mayonnaise, canned fruits

9. Vegetables

Stewed, steamed, boiled or raw

Creamed vegetables, soufflés, escalloped or au gratin

13. Staying on the Diet Long Enough to Get Thin—112 Useful Tips and Tricks to Conquer Compulsive Eating

On the following pages you will find 112 tips and tricks, separated into categories, to help you stay on your diet program. They are proven tactical strategies that help change the automatic eating habits that brought about your current need to lose weight. At the Health, Weight and Stress Program at Johns Hopkins we do not glamorize our handy hints gathered over many years for the use of our patients by calling them behavior modification techniques. They are simply useful tools—the majority, plain good common sense—though they may never have occurred to you before. Properly applied, they will help you eat in a more deliberate, controlled and aware manner.

Use the following strategies in the doses you need.

STRATEGIES FOR CONFRONTING AN ONCOMING BINGE

1. Binges are usually triggered by deprivation—overdieting—combined with stress. Low-carbohydrate diets are especially likely to bring on uncontrollable craving for sugars or starches because your body needs a certain amount of carbohydrate for energy.

   So the first strategy for confronting oncoming binges is to eat sensibly. Include a carbohydrate food at every meal. This does not mean candies and cakes, but fruits, grains, bread, pasta, potatoes, etc. Follow the University Medical Diet.

2. If you feel a binge coming on, put something *sour* in your mouth: a pickle, a slice of lemon or lime. Suck on it for a while. It affects your taste buds and may eliminate your current craving for sweets entirely.

3. If you absolutely can't resist something sweet, choose a flavorful fruit or juice or just the *tiniest* quantity necessary of a sugar food to get you through the crisis.

4. If your choice is fruit, don't gobble it down in a few bites. Take your time. Cut it up into small pieces, and sit down at the table to eat it with a fork.

5. Buy some low-calorie orange or grapefruit juice, worth only a few calories an ounce. Freeze it in molds for a quick fix when you feel yourself going up the wall.

6. Don't read this one unless your binge is totally out of control because it is unpleasant! Nevertheless, it works for many of our people when nothing else does. Here it is: Ask yourself what is the most revolting thing you could discover in the food you are eating—mold, a worm, a hairball, a dirty hand preparing the food, grease. Look at the food you are longing for, or think about it, and for three minutes imagine it this way. If you now decide to eat it, you are asking to be fat!

7. An unscheduled urge to stuff yourself? Take evasive action. Do something active that you really enjoy or need to accomplish, from exercise to knitting to taking a bath or scrubbing the floor. Talk on the telephone, or write a letter. Keep at it for at least half an hour, sipping water if you can to make you feel full.

8. Another way to outwit your urges: Brush your teeth with flavored toothpaste. If that's not sufficient, gargle and rinse your mouth with a strong mouthwash.

9. Keep "snowballs" in your freezer for the times you know you'll need a sweet taste. Make them out of crushed ice and diet soda, frozen in little paper cups or plastic bags. Eat them slowly with a small dessert spoon.

10. Suck on an ice cube. Bite it; crunch it; enjoy it.

11. Don't fool yourself that you're going to eat "just one" if you really know very well you are going to have another, and another, and another. If you never start, you won't have to finish.

12. Set a timer for ten minutes, and keep busy. When it goes off, ask yourself whether you are still truly hungry. If you are, go ahead and eat, but choose an *unfavorite* food with low calories.

13. Place a tablet of artificial sweetner on your tongue. Let it dissolve slowly.

14. Hungry? Starving? Dying for a Danish or a chicken leg, but mealtime is still a couple of hours away? Take a brisk walk or a bike ride. It will remove you from temptation, increase your metabolism and depress your appetite. Or try jogging in place, even more strenuous and effective.

15. Freeze it! If you are casting your eye on a delicious-looking piece of cake, a leftover pork chop, a roll that emits irresistible vibes to eat it, place it promptly in the freezer. When you finally take it out, you'll say to yourself, "Bless my good sense. That would have meant the road to disaster."

16. Remember that just *thinking* about how delicious a piece of pie or a slab of roast beef would taste (sorry!) can set off a chain of physiological responses that makes it extremely difficult to resist a binge. Can you feel it now? Is your mouth watering, and are your taste buds tingling? That's because if you are unduly influenced by environmental cues, the mere thought, sight or sound of food can turn you on, releasing a surge of insulin into your bloodstream. Quick! Deliberately turn your thoughts to another subject and force yourself to stick with it. If necessary, use the aversion technique described in number 6.

17. Or how about some frozen grapes? Store a bunch of seedless green grapes in the freezer, ready to pop into your mouth when you crave something sweet. Each one gives you only three little calories.

18. Some overweight people make regular middle-of-the-night raids on the kitchen and in the morning swear they have slept straight through the night. If you have this problem, hook up an alarm or bells to the refrigerator, and you'll be startled out of your sleepwalk before you can take a bite.

19. When you feel the urge to eat, polish your fingernails—two coats. They take time to dry.

STRATEGIES FOR THE HOMEFRONT

1. Get all X-rated foods out of your house. Why tempt fate? If they aren't there, you can't eat them, and a trip to the store takes conscious planning and execution. If you must have some for other members of the family (and usually they are better off without them, too), keep them out of sight and out of reach. Lock them away in a closet and give away the custody of the key, or store them in the garage. Put them on high shelves, their pictures turned to the rear. Make your refrigerator and kitchen cabinets as boring as possible—keep nothing there that lights up your eyes.

2. Store leftovers and other dangerous foods in individual portions in foil or covered opaque containers. Then push them to the back of the refrigerator so you won't be tempted to reach for the remains of last Saturday night's party when you open the door for an apple.

3. Cook just enough food to fill the plates just once. Don't plan for leftovers unless you're sure you can cope with their presence before you can make another meal of them.

4. Never serve family-style, placing bowls of food on the table. Instead, dole out the portions in the kitchen, and if other members of the family want seconds, let them go get them.

5. Tape-record mealtime conversations for a week or two. Quietly turn on the recorder at the start of each family meal; then listen to it later. Are your meals full of tension, strife, nagging? Do you eat at breakneck speed, eager to get it over with and on to the next activity? Can you hear yourself asking for the butter, the sugar, the gravy? Are you urged to have extra helpings, to break down and eat dessert because it's really delicious tonight and it's homemade? Does the family engage in real conversation, or is the concentration on food? Are the children included? Are the adults? Listening to the nuances at the table, decide if your way of eating is conducive to becoming a thin person. If it isn't, start changing the pattern.

6. Serve yourself meals on a small plate in a quiet, plain pastel color. Or choose gray, dark green, brown. These colors depress the appetite for many people. Avoid busy bright-colored patterns. Use small bowls for cereals, fruits, soups, desserts.

7. No naps! Overweight people get sleepy more often than thin people, though whether that's the result of their weight or its cause nobody knows. What we do know is that too much sleeping is fattening. Find something to do that intrigues you, preferably physical activity. A half hour's brisk walk will do you more good and will be more refreshing than a half hour's sleep.

8. Stay out of the kitchen. Enter it only when absolutely necessary.

Get Less Sleep

Shorten your nights! We have found in surveys of thousands of people in our weight-loss classes that **those who are overweight sleep, on the average, one to two and a third hours longer than thinner people.** Don't do it!

Try getting less sleep, and see if you don't feel just as good as or maybe a whole lot better than before. Most of us don't require more than six or seven or sometimes eight hours of sleep a night. Get up an hour earlier than usual, and spend the extra time doing something that keeps you moving. Take a bath, go for a walk, do your housework, exercise—anything is better for calorie consumption than lying in bed. Even sitting up to watch television burns more calories than sleeping.

Exception: This does not apply to you if you are already a short or poor sleeper, especially if you are a late-night eater.

---

9. Never go to the food market hungry. Shop after a satis-fying meal. Go only once a week, and stick to your list. No impulse buying. If necessary, take only a limited amount of cash with you to force you to hold the line.

10. Limit your exposure to table scraps. If you can, delegate the table clearing to somebody else. Or when you clear, scrape the plates immediately into the garbage pail; then place them promptly in the sink or dishwasher. Do not let scrap-laden plates remain in your presence for even a moment.

11. Another way to take the allure out of scraps: Throw them into the garbage pail, and empty your ashtrays or coffee grounds over them.

12. If you are a more resolute scrap eater, while you are still at the table, pour a hefty amount of salt over the left-overs.

13. Chew gum while you cook. To take a nibble, you must de-liberately remove it.

14. Or serve yourself a hot drink to diminish the need to taste and nibble.

15. Eat in only one place, at a table, sitting down. Eat every-thing, including snacks, from a plate, using a fork or spoon. Never take even a bite of food beyond the thresh-old of the kitchen or dining room. No food goes into the living room, bedroom, den or any other room in your house. Ever.

16. Does television whet your appetite? Keep your hands oc-cupied. Sew. Knit. Manicure your nails. Do home repairs. Whittle. Tie knots in string. Better yet, do some exercise in front of the set.

17. No eating while you drive. Concentrate on the road. Don't take snacks along for company.

18. Plan ahead if you are going to entertain at your home. First, remember that many of the people you know today are weight-conscious and would be delighted not to be faced with high-calorie temptation. But if you equate dinner parties with "fancy" food, for your own sake and

that of your guests, serve all gravies, dressings and sauces on the side. Always have some fruit for dessert, preferred by many people today, as an alternative to the more extravagant creations. You know how hard it is to resist pressure to eat the wrong foods or to accept more than your share. Don't pressure your guests!

19. Go out and buy yourself a pretty place mat and matching napkin. Every time you decide to eat, set the table attractively, and sit down to enjoy your food. Overeaters sometimes aren't even aware that they are eating, and this little ritual will force you to become conscious that you are.

20. Give your dining companions a head start—come to the table last. Let them start eating before you because you are probably a rapid eater who normally finishes quickly and then starts working on seconds. By coming late, you may finish on schedule.

21. If you are a late-night eater, take a glass of skim milk or a peeled and sectioned orange up to bed with you. Sip the milk or eat an orange segment when you feel the need to stuff.

STRATEGIES TO BOGGLE YOUR MIND

1. Faced by temptation, stand back for a minute. Ask yourself: "Do I want that lasagna *more* than I want to be thin?" If you answer the first part of the question in the affirmative, eat only a third of it.

2. An alternative approach: Visualize ten more pounds on your frame. Then add five more pounds and ask yourself, "Do I really want this food? Is it worth it? Will it make me gloriously happy at this moment and ten minutes from now?" And the opposite: Close your eyes, and imagine yourself as thin as you want to be. Then let that vision do the eating.

3. Post a favorite slim picture—of yourself or somebody else—in strategic places around the house. Don't forget the refrigerator door.

4. While you are on the program and losing weight, take a trip to the stores every couple of weeks and try on clothes. When you notice that you are beginning to fit into smaller and smaller sizes and that you are looking more attractive, it will give you motivation to make it down to the size you really want to be.

5. But don't *buy* clothes that are still too small for you. This is something many overweight people do, saying to themselves, "I'll fit into this in another month." We have found it can discourage you if you don't shed your excess pounds as fast as you fantasize.

6. Pick a psychologically compatible pal to diet with—if not your spouse, then a friend, a sibling, a colleague, somebody you spend a lot of time with or with whom you can be in constant touch. Share your problems and your triumphs; trade recipes; eat together; go on walks or bike trips instead of eating. Keep track of each other's progress; provide encouragement and an ear. The buddy system really helps if you don't get too competitive. There's an old saying, "There are no friends at an auction"; in this context, that means conscious or unconscious competition over the number of pounds lost can weaken a friendship.

7. Condition yourself: According to Dr. Peter Lindner, former president of The American Society of Bariatric Physicians, you can *practice* control. "Put your favorite kind of cake in front of you, and take a big forkful, bring it up to your mouth and say out loud, 'I can stop myself from eating this.' Then put the fork down. Do this ten times a day for a week. It helps."

8. Act thin. Pull your middle in, keep your shoulders back, and stride energetically. Don't wear "fat clothes"—baggy pants, overblouses, loose jackets. Tuck your shirt in; wear a belt; sit up straight so your waistband won't bind; wear clothes that *fit*—not baggy and not tight, but comfortable.

9. Watch another overweight person eat in a restaurant or cafeteria. Is it a pleasant sight? Is that how you look? Do

you want to look like that? Don't you feel a little superior when you order a superthin meal?

10. When you find yourself heading for the refrigerator or the cookie jar and you *know* you aren't physiologically hungry, give yourself a little psychotherapy: Sit down, close your eyes and contemplate. What emotions, tensions, problems, stresses are you feeling? Can you think of other ways to cope with them or distract you from them instead of eating?

11. "The devil made me do it"—the idea that something outside yourself that you can't control, that is overpowering you—has got to go. *You* are in control of yourself. Only you can pick up a spoon or a fork and feed yourself.

12. If you haven't found a "diet pal," ask a thin friend to call you every morning, to ask what you ate yesterday and what you plan to eat today. Don't discuss anything but your weight and your diet. Use this person as your therapist to support you through your diet program.

13. Avoid overweight friends if they make you feel skinny! It's too easy to delude yourself that you look great and it may remove your resolve.

14. Watch what thin and overweight people put into their shopping carts. It will help you realize that thin people aren't always born that way; they often help themselves along. They may be counting calories just as carefully as you are.

15. Reward yourself for losing weight. If you've done well, go out and buy yourself a little gift. Be honest. If you've been cheating, no reward. But don't reap your rewards in food—that spells disaster. Enlist your family in the reward system, too—they're close enough to you to praise you when you're doing well and to chide you when you are showing signs of fatigue.

16. When you get angry about being on a diet, let it all out! Most dieters feel frustrated and discouraged periodically, and you won't be an exception. Head for your bedroom,

and close the door. Punch your pillow hard over and over again, and shout, "I'm sick and tired of this ——— diet!"

17. Plan your weekends—but not around eating. Lots of dieters do fine from Monday through Friday, but weekends freak them out. Keep yourself busy, doing things you enjoy. It will keep your mind off food and away from the kitchen.

18. Forget the word *failure*. Being overweight is not a failure; it simply means you need to diet. Nor is it a failure if you go off your diet occasionally; it simply means you have to be more careful in the future.

19. Each morning make a fresh resolution that you will stick with your diet, *no matter what*.

20. Take a mind trip. Learn to relax and rid yourself of tensions and stress. Try one of our relaxation techniques.

STRATEGIES TO KEEP FROM "PIGGING OUT"

1. About half an hour before a meal take the edge off your hunger by drinking a tall glass of water. If it helps, add a teaspoon of artificial sweetener or a slice of lemon. Sip it slowly, and it will give you a noncaloric first course that will dispose you to eat less at the table. Occasionally, just for a change, try a low-calorie soda instead.

2. Consume as few calories as possible in liquid form because they won't be as satisfying as solid food and go down too easily. Avoid alcohol and wine, both full of calories, and regular soft drinks, which are like drinking flavored water with eight teaspoons of sugar added. Choose water, skim milk, bouillon, tomato juice, diet drinks instead.

3. If you eat a salad before you begin your meal, you can take the steam out of your appetite. Or chew celery stalks, cucumber sticks, carrots, or drink a glass of tomato juice, to satisfy your hunger so you don't become overly enthusiastic about the foods coming up. Eat your salad very cold, with a low-calorie dressing or lemon juice.

4. Or eat backward. Have some of your dessert *first*. If this works for you, the carbohydrate content will give you a quick lift and make you feel fuller at the start of the meal.

5. Always weigh or measure your portions. It often isn't *what* you eat, but *how much of it*, that adds up the calories. If you don't allot yourself a specific portion, it is much too easy to keep right on eating.

6. Concentrate not only on appearance, color, caloric content, nutrition and flavor but also on texture. If your food is rich in texture and takes some effort from your jaw muscles, it seems to go much further. Raw vegetables are a good choice. Another is unbuttered popcorn, which is virtually devoid of calories.

7. If you find yourself wanting to eat more than you know you should, get up from the table, go to the bathroom, and do the toothbrushing trick. Be sure to use a toothpaste with strong flavor. It soothes the craving that certain foods, especially sweet flavors, seem to create.

8. Have a pitcher of ice water on the table. Drink some with your meal.

9. Never allow yourself to become ravenous before you sit down to eat, or you'll definitely overeat. You'll eat faster, more, and taste the food less. Apply one of the tips we've already mentioned for taking the edge off your appetite, or make a habit of having a scheduled snack between meals.

10. If you do become overeager to eat, force yourself to wait for twenty minutes. Many people find that the urge to eat diminishes greatly if they hold out for a while.

11. Do you suffer from the old hang-up of scraping your plate clean? Even though Mom used to insist that you finish every bite, don't. Always leave something on your plate, even just a scrap, as a tangible sign to yourself that you can quit when you choose.

12. Eat with a cocktail fork, an idea thought up by one of our patients at Johns Hopkins and copied by almost every diet clinic in the country.

13. Don't try to give up all your most favorite foods, even if they are full of calories, because you may go wild with frustration and forget the whole diet. Just eat *less* of them. Ration yourself some servings of ice cream, if that's what you crave, or make a special occasion of spaghetti and meat sauce every couple of weeks. But always keep a record of it, and be sure the number of calories is within your total allowance, cutting back on other foods to make room for the specials.

14. Schedule your meals at fixed times every day, and stick to your routine as rigidly as you can: breakfast at seven thirty, lunch at twelve, dinner at six thirty, for example. Your between-meal cravings will diminish as you reeducate your body to healthy eating patterns.

15. Turn off the television set and the radio. Put every morsel of food you are going to eat—including snacks—on a plate. Sit down at your designated dining spot, and concentrate on *what* you are eating and *how* you are eating it. Never eat anywhere else. No nibbling out of a box in the kitchen. No bolting a glass of milk on your way out the door. No grabbing a carrot stick or a slice of meat on the run. Go to your table with every morsel of food or sip of a drink; sit down; eat or drink it *consciously*.

STRATEGIES ON THE WORKFRONT

1. If it's not easy getting what you need for lunch in restaurants and cafeterias, brown-bag your lunch. This way you have food that conforms to your own plan. Pack salads and low-calorie desserts in plastic containers. Take cans of water-packed tuna fish or salmon or even vegetables, and don't forget a can opener. Use a small thermos for hot soup or cold drinks. You'll not only have an easier time staying on your diet but save a tremendous amount of money.

2. Don't eat at your desk. If the weather is good, find an attractive place outdoors for a picnic. At least change your location in your building before you open your lunch bag.

3. Beware of imitation milk products like nondairy creamers. They are usually loaded with sugar or fat. Ask for a
   little plain milk for your coffee.

4. The coffee break, the great American pastime, is dangerous, a menace to any diet program. Take an exercise break
   instead. Go for a walk, a run, or do calisthenics. If you find
   a buddy to do it with you, that helps. If you can't resist
   joining your colleagues at the table, always be prepared
   with your own snacks from home—a hard-boiled egg, a
   piece of fruit, cheese, melba toast. Remember to count
   them among your exchanges.

5. In your desk keep an emergency ration of foods that you
   like well enough but that don't turn you on and, of course,
   are low-calorie. They can keep you from raiding the
   vending machines. Suggestions: water-packed canned
   fish, instant broth or boullion, water chestnuts, dill pickles, instant iced tea, vegetables, fruit. Be sure to account
   for them in your total food plan.

6. When you go out for lunch, try a delicatessen where the
   meat can be weighed in the exact amount you request.
   Easy to ask for "three ounces of roast beef on rye."

7. Pick your eating companions. Don't go out to lunch with
   friends who can—and do—eat anything and never gain
   weight unless you can successfully resist the foods they
   eat. Dine with people who won't make you covet what's
   on their plates.

SLOWDOWN STRATEGIES

1. Never finish a meal in less than twenty minutes. That's
   how long it takes for the physiological signals of satiety to
   travel from your stomach to your brain. That's a scientific
   fact. Savor your meal, chew every bite thoroughly, concentrate on what you are eating and, when you are finished, you will be much more satisfied with your portions.
   If necessary, take a short break mid-meal before you have
   dessert. People who gulp their food usually poke around,
   looking for a little more of this or that. In an hour or two

after a meal they're "hungry" again. Besides, if you eat fast, you are much more likely to eat *more* of everything simply because you don't realize you have had enough.

2. Cut your food into very small pieces, pick them up with your fork and put them into your mouth one by one. If necessary, use a pair of chopsticks. Unless you are an Oriental, it's impossible to eat fast with a couple of skinny sticks. Or use the cocktail fork, especially for foods like spaghetti.

3. Use a two-minute timer. Eat for two minutes. Rest for two minutes. Think about how the food is filling you up. Then start again.

4. Put only one food in your mouth at a time. Don't mix everything or anything together with another food—on your plate or on your fork. No more mouthfuls until you have swallowed the last. You'll be surprised how much more you enjoy your food.

5. Never gulp liquids. Sip them slowly, savoring the taste.

6. Place your utensils on your plate after every third mouthful. Wait at least thirty seconds before picking them up again while you concentrate on something other than food. Conversation perhaps?

7. Chew each mouthful at least ten times if it is soft food and up to twenty times if it is chewy or crunchy. Remember to count.

8. Eat to enjoy your food. Pay attention to the taste and the texture, the quality of the food. Is it sweet? Spicy? Can you identify the seasonings? Does it remind you of other times, other places? Take your time and use this opportunity to become a gourmet instead of a gobbler.

9. Prop a big mirror in front of you so that you get an unobstructed view of your mouth, and watch yourself eat. Is it an attractive sight? Are you shoveling the food in, overstuffing your face? A few sessions with the mirror can break you of speed eating if you remember what you have seen.

10. Choose foods that aren't too easy to cope with. For example, take chicken pieces rather than boneless chicken breast; eat corn on the cob instead of corn kernels, whole fruits, unshelled nuts. Rather than soft, creamy foods that slide down without effort, pick foods that require chewing, biting, crunching.

11. Use a utensil—a knife, fork, spoon—to eat everything, even bread, bananas, crackers.

STRATEGIES FOR PARTIES, RESTAURANTS, VACATIONS

1. When you are going to a gathering where you know food will be the focus, eat some safe foods before you go so you won't walk in ravenous, devouring the hors d'oeuvres as you pass through the door. Have a slice of bread, some fruit or vegetables, a big glass of water.

2. Don't get there early. Hold off until you know the party will be well under way. Leave early, too, to get yourself out of the way of temptation.

3. Here are a few other ways of handling social gatherings, all of which have worked for some of our members. Take your choice: (1) Turn down all invitations until you have reached your diet goal; (2) stick to carrot sticks and celery stalks, or eat nothing at all; (3) eat the hors d'oeuvres—but skip dinner afterward.

4. If a special occasion is on the calendar, plan ahead. If you know you are certain to overeat this Saturday night, put some calories in the bank. A couple of hundred calories saved every day from Monday through Friday will give you leeway. For example, skip dessert on Monday, a piece of bread on Tuesday, a snack on Wednesday. But *remember:* This is only a once-in-a-while arrangement. You can't do it every week, or your diet plan will rapidly founder. This doesn't mean you can eat everything in sight; it just means you are about 1,000 calories to the good and needn't be so uptight about your diet on *that one evening.*

Warning: Many people can't cope with this concept, because it gives them license to overindulge. To use this tip, you must be able to keep an accurate count of calories (and exchanges) and use the count to your advantage.

5. You can put some calories in escrow, saving them up ahead of time, for a vacation or the holiday season, too. For a few weeks before, cut back to give yourself some room to expand. When you have accumulated a few thousand banked calories (at 200 a day for four weeks, you have saved almost 6,000), you can spend them (or not) when the time comes. If you can hold back, you've lost almost a couple of pounds. Don't try this trick, however, unless you *know* you won't overspend your saved-up calories. It can be dangerous.

   When the vacation or the holidays are over, no malingering! Back to business and the program the very same day.

   By the way, never, never do it the other way around. If you plan to make up for overeating *after* the event, cutting down after going wild, you will rarely succeed. Some staunch people can do it, but we have found that very few dedicated overeaters can manage to make up for lost opportunities with ease.

6. Beware of buffet tables, which are a dieter's downfall. Such a big selection of tempting foods commands you to try everything maybe two or three times, especially since you eat standing up and tend to clean your plate in a hurry. Choose the *three* items you like best. Serve yourself small portions. And eat them *slowly.*

7. Salad bars, too, can be a problem. Salad sounds thinning, but it isn't if you cover it with high-calorie dressings and all the fattening little tidbits that accompany it, such as bacon bits, anchovies, olives, avocados, chickpeas, croutons, nuts. So pile on the lettuce and other greens; but avoid the wrong toppings, and flavor it with low-calorie dressing or just a little vinegar or lemon juice plus seasonings.

8. When you have a dinner party at home, if you know you'll be dipping into the leftovers when you shouldn't, give them all to the guests as they leave. Tell your friends they

are doing you an enormous favor by getting them out of your sight.

9. In a restaurant be the first to order so you won't be tempted to say, "That sounds good. I'll have that, too," to a meal that is not suitable for you.

10. Order your salad immediately. It will give you something to nibble on while you're waiting for your order to arrive.

11. Before a meal out, decide whether or not you are going to eat the bread and butter. If you make up your mind, "Yes, I am going to have bread," take your allotment; then move the bread basket to the opposite side of the table out of your reach, or ask the waiter to take it away.

12. Commit yourself publicly. Announce to your dinner companions exactly what you are going to eat. It will help you adhere to your plan.

13. Wear clothes, a belt, a girdle that are a little snug on you. Not much—you don't want to be uncomfortable or look stuffed into your clothes—but just enough so that when you have eaten your allowed allotment, you will be conscious of your expanded midsection.

14. In the early stages of your new diet program, call your hosts (if you know them well) before you go to a dinner party, and ask what's on the menu. If it's a dish you can't have, ask if you may bring something for yourself to be served with the meal.

15. Don't be intimidated by the waiter in a restaurant. Ask for what you want—meat or fish broiled without butter, salad dressing on the side or just a wedge of lemon, no sauce on the vegetables. The waiter is being paid (and tipped) to serve you what you want, not what is easiest for him to bring forth.

16. And don't be timid about asking for a "doggy bag" to take leftovers home—*if* they will make another meal (and not an unscheduled binge) for you. Even the best restaurants are used to such requests. You are paying for this food. It is yours.

17. Choose a restaurant that serves a variety of items and doesn't specialize in fried foods and heavy sauces. While you order, drink a low-calorie soda or a glass of water, and eat your salad. Choose your main course first, avoiding all the known pitfalls like breaded or fried foods and fatty meats. If the portions are very large, decide before you eat a bite just *how much* you are going to eat. Move the rest to another plate, and give it away or ask the waiter to remove it. Or perhaps you can arrange to share a dish with somebody else in your group. Big portions are no bargain if they make you fat.

18. If you know a "complete dinner" is going to be too much for you, order à la carte, ordering only what you want.

19. Resort hotels present problems because the rates often include meals and the average person wants his or her money's worth. Try all the tips and tricks we have recommended to keep you from feeling ravenous, and remember you don't have to go wild on this vacation unless you want to bring home a memento of ten or fifteen pounds. Decide beforehand what and how much you're going to eat. Use this opportunity to get added exercise—play golf, get into the volleyball game, take nice long hikes, swim. Don't just sit around the terrace or the swimming pool, sipping planter's punch.

14. Burning Off the Fat: Exercises for the Reluctant Athlete

Those people who jog and bike and live on the racquetball courts must be punishing themselves. Why do they want to suffer like that? It's definitely not for me. Tell the truth, I don't really get much exercise. It's hard enough working, taking care of the house, looking after the kids. Besides, exercise was never fun to me.

—Bookkeeper, female, age 33

When I was a kid, I was into sports. In college I played football, and for a while afterward I was pretty active. But now I don't do much, and I guess that's the reason for all this weight I've accumulated. I'm always making plans to start running or playing squash or something, but I never seem to have the time. I don't feel as good as I did when I was more active and thin.

—Forty-four-year-old engineering manager

If you are more than twenty pounds overweight, it is almost certain you don't get much exercise. **Most overweight people consider exercise a dirty word, a total turnoff and as a group, avoid moving their bodies more than necessary.** In our surveys of our weight classes we have found that less than 5 percent get *any* kind of regular exercise whatsoever. And every day? Forget it!

Not only do most perennially heavy people have a decided bias against physical activity, but they also exert as little effort as possible going about their everyday lives. Study after study has shown that, whatever they do, they do it *less* than thinner people do.

Though an estimated 55 million people in the United States today are participating in a fitness frenzy, it's doubtful you are. You may have joined an exercise class or bought a tennis racket and a new pair of shorts, but after an early flurry of activity your major form of exercise undoubtedly, once again, is watching the football games on television or climbing into your car.

THE MAJOR CAUSE OF FAT: SITTING DOWN

The truth is, however, that lack of exercise may well be the primary reason that the food you eat tends to stick to your ribs. And the single most effective way to lose it is to start moving that reluctant body.

In fact, if you have a lot of weight to lose, exercise may be the *only* way you can burn a sufficient number of calories without an overly stringent diet that you cannot continue to follow forever. It's the best way, too, to lower your set point effectively (see Chapter 5) so your body won't automatically return to its former weight after a significant loss.

Yes, you *can* lose weight without exercise. You can simply cut back on your food and never take one unnecessary step. But if you have already been eating low-calorie food, you are going to be *hungry.* You are going to feel deprived. And before too long you are likely to become discouraged and revert to your old ways and weight. That's because you are not helping yourself burn up calories fast. You have stacked the deck against yourself.

Some very overweight people *cannot* lose enough weight with diet alone. As a result of weighing too much too long, dieting too drastically, yoyoing back and forth between fat and thin, their metabolism slows down so much that they require remarkably few calories to maintain themselves in their overweight state. They may eat even fewer calories a day than a normal thin person. For them, exercise is not only important, but essential, if they want to lose weight, because it causes a compensatory metabolic rise.

HOW TO LOSE FASTER

When you increase your physical activity, you need not reduce your food intake drastically before you see a real difference on the scale. For example, if you decide to cut back 500 calories a day (3,500 a week, the equivalent of one pound), simply step up your exercise by a mere 250 calories and cut your food by 250 calories. You will lose weight faster and more easily since the combination adds up to more benefit than each one separately. And you'll have an important added feature: better health.

SPEEDING UP YOUR METABOLISM

Exercise, if it is vigorous enough, pays off, not once but *twice*. It makes your body burn up more calories while you are at it, but it does more than that: It alters your body chemistry, speeding up your metabolism so that after you have stopped, even while you sleep, your body continues for many hours to burn up the calories up to 20 percent more rapidly than normal. So even while you're sitting in your favorite chair, watching television, your body is still busily burning extra calories as the result of an afternoon workout.

After a vigorous exercise session your metabolic rate may remain elevated for one to twenty-four hours. The increased caloric expenditure results from the body's need to dissipate heat and to restore the tissues after hard use. An added attraction: By revving up your metabolism, exercise makes you feel more energetic. This encourages you to exercise even more. As you increase your muscle tissue through regular exercise, you'll burn even more calories because muscle requires more calories to maintain than fat does.

BONUS: Exercise is also said to help ward off infectious illnesses, according to a study sponsored by the National Institute of General Medical Sciences at the University of Michigan. By speeding up metabolism and therefore your generation of body heat, it acts just like a fever as a natural defense mechanism. The higher body temperature—which lasts several hours after a vigorous workout—and the increased number of infection-fighting white blood cells in circulation produce an environment that is hostile to bacteria. That's why, exercisers claim, they get sick less often than armchair athletes.

"BUT EXERCISE WILL MAKE ME HUNGRY!"

Wrong. That is a myth. **Exercise won't make you hungry. It will help you enjoy your food more, but it won't make you eat more. In fact, vigorous exercise suppresses appetite for thirty minutes to an hour after you have stopped. It is a temporary appetite depressant.**

A good strategy: Plan a five- to ten-minute session of moderate exercise—a brisk walk, dancing, calisthenics, etc.—ending five minutes before a meal. It will help curb your appetite.

EXERCISE RAISES YOUR SPIRITS

Exercise is also an excellent psychological stimulant that doesn't involve drugs or even a cup of coffee. It relieves boredom and depression, thereby removing some of the major reasons you may be overeating. It reduces tension. Most overweight people, we have discovered, have a high level of anxiety. This decreases demonstrably after only two weeks of physical exercise.

Exercise that increases your heart rate and expands your lungs can produce a physiological "high," and you needn't turn into a dedicated jogger to experience it. By triggering the release of beta endorphin, a morphinelike substance secreted by the brain, as well as other mood-elevating natural chemicals, it produces a feeling of euphoria and well-being.

ANTIFLAB TREATMENT

If you do not combine diet with regular exercise, you can count on flab. No diet plan ever devised, no matter what anyone claims, will especially prevent sags and bags, if you lose more than ten or twenty pounds and are over thirty-five or forty years old. **The only lasting antidote is exercise,** most effective the younger you are, but helpful at any age. It will tone your muscles, firm you up. An increase in lean body mass (muscle) while you are losing fat will definitely give your skin a more taut appearance. And even at the same weight, you will look trimmer because muscle tissue has a much smaller volume than fat.

The potential for flab is a good reason not to try a high-protein crash diet, because along with losing fat tissue, you will lose muscle tissue, the part of you that gives you shape. You may end up thinner, but you will have lost your muscle resilience. You will end up looking gaunt and haggard as well as saggy.

THE MORE YOU WEIGH, THE MORE YOU LOSE!

Good news for the overweight population! **If you're very much overweight, your weight loss from exercise is much quicker than**

it is for thinner people. If you are a 250-pounder who exercises with a friend, a 125-pounder, you will burn more calories in the same amount of time and with the same effort. That means you will lose more weight. (By the way, the taller you are, the more calories you consume in the same time and with the same effort, too.)

But there is a catch. As you reduce your body's fat content, you may have to adjust your equation because with a smaller body to nourish, you will now burn *fewer* calories doing the same thing.

BUT IS IT WORTH IT?

Are you saying to yourself, "But I've heard you have to walk thirty-five miles or play tennis for six hours to burn off a pound of fat! So what's the use?"

It doesn't work that way. Every small amount of physical activity you add to your daily schedule is cumulative. It all adds up. You don't have to walk thirty-five miles at one time or stay on the court until you drop. Just increase your expenditure here and there, wherever you can, and it will add up to hundreds of calories that won't be transformed into fat.

EXERCISE IS A PIECE OF CAKE

No matter how much you have revved yourself up to start a diet and lose weight, you may not stick to it more than a couple of weeks if you have to force yourself to exercise. So the first thing to do is change your attitude about it. Being a little more physical needn't mean you must become an athlete.

If you haven't exercised in years, even the smallest increase will quickly make a difference. Simply standing instead of sitting, and walking instead of standing, use more energy. It's been estimated that the energy cost of standing or walking for a very heavy person is four times that of sitting! Bending over is exercise. Climbing stairs is exercise. Moving your arms up and down or kicking your feet in the bathtub is exercise. You can do it. You do it now. Just do it *more,* and do it *faster.* Start weaving body movements into your daily existence, and they will soon add up to a lot of calories.

Using the methods taught at our clinic, begin with activities you can do easily. And remember, there's no harm in being a closet exerciser if you're self-conscious.

DOES IT FEEL LIKE EXERCISE?

What kind of exercise speeds up metabolism and burns up the most calories? The very same kind that strengthens your cardiovascular system. It's the kind that *feels* like exercise. It raises your heart rate. It expands your lungs. It consumes more oxygen. It involves the body's large muscles, moving in a continuous and repetitive pattern. Metabolism-raising activity requires some exertion, some effort, makes you sweat a little. And to get maximum benefit, you must push yourself—not much, just a little—increasing your efforts gradually over a period of time.

We don't recommend that you strain yourself, become exhausted, huff and puff and make yourself dizzy, because that is not good for you and it will not encourage you to continue. You don't have to take up aerobic dancing or jogging through the streets at 6:00 A.M. especially since, as an exercise hater, you won't keep it up. But it means you can't be satisfied with raising your pinkie to lift a teacup or even taking a leisurely walk in the park. You require enough exertion to encourage a deficit in calories.

If you're out of condition and especially if you are very much overweight, walking may be your best option. It's one of the most oxygen-burning (aerobic) exercises you can do, believe it or not, if you move right along. It is in moving the most weight (your whole self) the greatest distance that you burn the most calories. Another excellent exercise for which you need no lessons is stair climbing. Researchers at the University of Pennsylvania estimate an overweight person can lose ten to twelve pounds a year just by climbing an additional two flights of stairs a day.

HOW MUCH, HOW OFTEN?

This is the hitch for the most reluctant exercisers. If you want to lose weight at your optimum rate, you must exercise at least three times a week for at least half an hour each time.

MAKE IT EASY FOR YOURSELF

In our weight-loss clinic, participants learn exercises that they practice in class, then continue at home. Instructed by Hyland Levasseur, our exercise consultant, a faculty member, and a representative of the President's Council on Physical Fitness, they quickly progress at their own levels of achievement. You can do the same.

If you are extremely overweight, note the special section for you starting on page 224.

Remember the cardinal rules:

1. Get your doctor's permission before starting on any exercise program because even the mildest forms of activities can be harmful for some people.

2. Always start slowly, gradually working up to your maximum exertion.

3. Stop when you feel any strain or stress.

Spot Reducing: Can It Be Done?

Forget spot reducing. There is no such thing. You cannot change your basic body build or specific areas of your body by exercise, diet, machines, hot packs, massage or any other way. You can simply get thinner all over, perhaps with the most weight lost in the areas of greatest concentration.

No gadget or manipulation can shift fat tissue from one part of the body to another or even reduce it. In fact, some studies have shown that massage, by improving local circulation, may stimulate the fat cells in the area to accumulate *more* fat. And research on belt vibrators proved these gadgets are useless.

You can, however, tone and firm specific parts of your body through exercise so they will be more shapely and so look slimmer.

GETTING THE MOST OUT OF EXERCISE

1. Consult your body clock. Schedule your exercise for the times of day when your resistance to food temptation is at its low ebb. This way you will be doing something else at a moment when you might otherwise be stuffing food into your mouth, and you will be taking an appetite-depressant "pill." If you're a Night Eater, for example, exercise in the evening to take the edge off your cravings. If you normally snack in the afternoons, turn your coffee break into an exercise break. For most people, afternoons are the time physical ability is at its peak.

2. Exercising in a cold temperature burns more calories. That's because you need energy to maintain normal body temperature and carry around heavy clothing. Even your basal metabolism is higher when it's cold. So use cold weather to your advantage—get out there and move. At home, turn the thermostat down or open the window. You will make your own heat and lose more weight.

3. Though heavy exercise is not recommended after meals, studies show that a half hour of light exercise after meals doubles the energy expended and dramatically decreases fat storage. A five- to ten-minute warm-up before your main meal of the day and a moderate thirty-minute session afterward looks like your best bet, so get up from the table and take the dog for a walk!

FOR SIX-SECOND INTERVALS

You can fit some quick exercise into the little intervals in your life. For example:

· Stand up or pace around while you're talking on the telephone.

· At work, click your heels together or kick your legs up and down under your desk. Flexing your feet helps.

· Run in place as you wait for the toaster to pop or the TV commercial to end. Do a couple of deep knee bends when you're picking something off the floor.

· Standing in line at the supermarket, take a deep breath, draw your shoulders back, pull your stomach in and tighten your buttocks. Hold it. Then relax. Repeat a few times.

· Waiting in traffic for a light to change, flatten your abdomen from groin to rib cage. Hold it; relax; repeat as many times as you can.

· Lying in bed in the morning, flat on your back, place your hands under your head, and lift it against the resistance of your neck muscles. Lift until your chin touches your chest; then lower your head slowly. Now repeat, and lift your shoulders as well.

· Stand up to put on your shoes, leaning against a wall if necessary.

· Sitting in a chair, bounce up and down as many times as you can, using your leg muscles for lift.

· Sitting near a wall, lift your feet and push your heels forward as if you were trying to push the wall away, raising your toes so you feel the muscles in the backs of your legs pulling like a rope. Count to six, and slowly relax.

Remember that your small investments of exercise total up to a nice dividend by the end of the day.

EXERCISES FOR NONATHLETES: PLAN 1

If you are not accustomed to doing much more than walking over to the refrigerator and opening the door, you cannot begin a vigorous exercise program without working up to it very gradually, especially if you are very much overweight. So start by doing the following series of exercises, which you will eventually use as warm-ups for more strenuous sessions. It should take about twenty minutes to complete. This series was originated for the Health, Weight and Stress Program at Johns Hopkins by Agnes M. Taylor of the Maryland Commission on Physical Fitness.

Starter Warm-ups

1. Deep Breathing

Take deep breath; rise on toes with arms extended over head; exhale slowly, lowering arms slowly. Repeat three times.

2. Walk in Place

Lift left knee up; then lower knee. Lift right knee up; then lower knee. Repeat ten times.

3. Arm Swings

Swing right arm, rotating forward, five times. Reverse motion, rotating backward, five times. Repeat with left arm. With both arms together in a windmill fashion, swing forward five times. Reverse five times.

4. Finger Squeeze

Extend arms shoulder height in front, palms down. Squeeze the fingers slowly; then release. Repeat five times. Then turn palms up; squeeze fingers five times. Extend arms again in front, and shake fingers five times.

5. Arm Turns

Extend arms to the side, palms up. Cup hands, turn arms down in a circular movement and return to starting position. Repeat five times.

6. Shoulder Rolls

Beginning with elbows bent and to your sides, roll shoulders forward in full circle, slowly, five times. Reverse by rolling shoulders backward in a circle, slowly, five times. Arms down at your sides, shrug shoulders up and down, five times.

7. Body Stretch

Extend right foot forward as far as it will go, bending your knee, leaving the left foot firmly planted. Bend body forward with arms extended over your bent knee. Stretch forward five counts, stretching farther forward on each count. Reverse procedure. Lift up on your toes; stretch overhead to count of five.

8. Head and Neck Exercise

Place hands on hips; bend head forward so that chin touches the chest. Now bend head backward as far as it will go; then bend head to starting position, and turn the head to the left; return head to starting position, and then turn head to the right. Repeat five times.

9. Body Bends and Turns

Place hands on hips. Slowly bend your body forward at the waist as far as it will go; then bend body back. Return body to starting position. Keep hips facing forward; turn upper torso to the left. Return to starting position, and turn upper body to the right. Repeat five times.

10. Body Side Stretch

Place left hand on left hip, extending right arm over head. Bend to left side toward the ground, to the count of two. Return to starting position, place right hand on right hip, with left arm extended upward over head, and bend to the right, to the count of two.

11. Posture Exercise

Stand erect with feet about six inches apart. Tighten leg muscles; tighten stomach by drawing it in. Extend chest, bring arms up, elbows out to sides, clenched fists chest-high. Take deep breath; let it out slowly (keeping the muscles taut and rigid), vibrating arms back for a count of three.

12. Arm Thrusts

Stand with feet six inches apart. Make fists, bend elbows next to your body. Thrust arms forward; bring back. Thrust them sideward; bring back; then upward and down. Repeat three times.

EXERCISES FOR NONATHLETES: PLAN 2

After two or three weeks of the starter warm-ups, move along to a slightly more strenuous set of moves planned by Hyland Levasseur. These simple exercises can be easily done even by people who have a lot of weight to lose. Begin by going through each exercise only three or four times, and work up to ten repetitions. End each by returning to the starting position. Stop and breathe deeply after each exercise. If any of the exercises seems too difficult or too strenuous for you, *stop* as soon as you feel any strain. Exercise for at least a half hour each session after you have reached ten repetitions. You will become more limber and agile and ready to move on to more strenuous metabolism-raising sessions that will help you lose weight faster.

Do the deep breathing exercise (number 1 of starter warm-ups) before beginning and after finishing each exercise session.

Intermediate Simple Exercises

1. Stutter Steps

Jump, simultaneously bringing the left foot forward and the right foot to the rear. Jump again, bringing the right foot forward and the left foot to the rear. Now jump three more times in quick succession, reversing the position of the feet each time. The entire exercise includes five jumps in each of four directions: front, left, rear and right.

2. Leg Huggers

Raise right knee as high as possible, grasping leg with both hands and pulling your knee into the body. Lower, and repeat with left leg.

3. Hop-Jumps

Jump, simultaneously moving feet sideward and apart in a single motion; then spring back to the starting position. Now hop on the left foot and then on the right foot.

4. Forward Crawl Stroke

Right leg forward, arms at sides, bend slightly forward at the waist, rotate arms alternately in large circles from the shoulder joints, similar to the crawl stroke in swimming. Repeat with left leg forward.

5. Side-to-Side Stretch

With feet a comfortable distance apart and arms outstretched overhead, bend as far to the right and then to the left as far as possible.

6. Hands-on-Shoulders Knee Lifts

Start with hands on shoulders. Bring the left knee up and the right elbow down to meet each other. Return to starting position. Then bring the right knee up and left elbow down to meet each other.

7. Overhead Circles

Stand with feet a comfortable foot apart, both arms stretched straight overhead as far as possible without rising to your toes, spreading your fingers wide apart. Rotate arms and entire upper body in unison in a circular motion. Each complete circle counts as one repetition.

8. Step Squats

Stand with hands on hips. Take a large step forward with right foot, squat down and touch the left knee to the floor. Now return to starting position. Repeat with the left foot forward.

9. The Airplane

Stand with legs wide apart; bend forward with arms extended sideward at shoulder height, palms down; now pull arms backward, slowly rotating the arms backward and upward until the palms are up.

10. Bend to Allah

With feet spread and hands overhead, bend back; then touch hands to floor in front.

11. Elbow Touches and Lifts

Start with hands on shoulders, elbows out to the side. Bring the elbows forward, and touch; then lift elbows straight upward as far as possible.

12. Bend and Reach

Start with legs wide apart, hands on hips. Bend and reach with both hands toward the left foot, twice to the center front and then to the right foot. Return to starting position.

13. Arm Rotations

Beginning with right arm, make the widest possible circle to the front; reverse. Repeat with left arm. Then, bending slightly backward, use both arms to make circles forward. Reverse.

14. Bent-Over Windmill

Start with legs wide apart. Bend over so that back is parallel to the floor with arms outstretched at shoulder height. Simultaneously swing left arm down and right arm back as far as possible. Repeat with the right arm down and left arm back.

15. Cross-Over Toe Touches

Start at attention. Cross left leg over the right. Stretch twice with both hands toward the right foot. Repeat with right leg crossed over the left, stretching twice with both hands toward the left foot.

16. Jog in Place

With forearms held about waist high, body erect, jog in place for one minute. Gradually work up to five minutes, increasing one minute per week.

EXERCISES FOR SEMIATHLETES: PLAN 3

If you are a real athlete, you don't need our help. You'll be out there, rain or shine, jogging, dancing, playing a swift game of singles, without prodding from weight-loss experts.

Nonathletes who have mastered Plans 1 and 2 are now advised to graduate to Plan 3, exercises that will speed up their metabolisms and take the pounds off quickly. Recommended here are several varieties of easy-to-do aerobic exercises to raise your heart rate, increase your lung expansion and burn up more calories. Heroics are not required or even desirable. Start out with a program you can manage without strain, and build up gradually until you are doing your maximum for at least a half hour every other day.

Monitor your pulse rate: Before you begin any strenuous exercise session, including the ones outlined here, count your pulse rate at rest. Then count it again after five or ten minutes of exercise, at least for the first two weeks. Never continue to exercise if the rate exceeds your target range.

Here's how to monitor your pulse: Place your thumb and first two fingers on either side of your throat just below your jawbone. Here you can feel the pulsing of your carotid arteries. Using a watch with a second hand, count your heart beats for ten seconds. Multiply by six for the count for one minute. When you take your pulse during or after your exercise session, count it *immediately* after stopping, within a couple of seconds. Heart rate slows down very rapidly when you rest.

Your desirable increase: There is a simple and generally accepted formula for calculating an oxygen-consuming or aerobic heart rate: Take the number 220; subtract your age; then figure out 75 percent of that number. For example, if you are forty years old, your pulse rate should probably not exceed 134. If you are fifty, it shouldn't go beyond 128.

Walking.

This is the best all-around exercise for everyone simply because it requires nothing more than a good pair of shoes. It's safe, and it's easy. It involves all the major muscles of the body, it can be done at any level of energy, it can provide the very same health benefits as jogging and it fits easily into a daily routine. Another advantage: It doesn't leave you exhausted, though it is just as beneficial as more strenuous activities.

By walking, we do not mean strolling in a leisurely fashion around the garden, smelling the flowers. You must keep up a brisk, businesslike pace, moving along speedily enough so that when you eventually reach your peak performance, you can cover three miles in an hour.

If you are very overweight and/or very sedentary, forget miles. Think in terms of one block. Start off slowly, visualizing pulling a little red cart behind you loaded with maybe twenty-five or fifty or seventy-five pounds more than the average person. Let the distance be your guide. Take it slowly; take it safely and sanely. Then gradually increase both your distance and your speed as you feel comfortable doing it.

Before long you can work up to a minimum of a half hour. Walk briskly so that you breathe deeply but can still keep up a conversation. Go as fast as you can, without stopping to window-shop, chat with your neighbors, or do errands. The idea is to be vigorous, pushing yourself a little more each time, breathing a little harder, going a little farther than you think you can, for half an hour at least every other day.

Check your pulse before starting, then again in ten minutes. If your heart rate is too high, stop to rest or slow down. If it's too low, try to pick up your pace.

If you walk for fifteen minutes a day, as briskly as you can, you can achieve a weight loss of up to twenty-six pounds in a year— and that's on a maintenance diet. Together with a diet that gives you a 300-calorie deficit a day, you can lose more than fifty pounds in only a year.

Swimming.

This is another excellent all-around exercise that provides everything you need. It gets your heart rate up there where you want it and moves all your major muscles. It's a complete exercise, giving you the same benefits as jogging, for example, though it is much easier because the buoyancy of the water takes the stress off your joints.

As with all the other choices, regularity and exerting yourself more and more as you become more fit are the keys. Remember, if exercise is going to accomplish its maximum calorie-burning feats, it must *feel* like exercise. Swim continuously, gradually increasing your endurance until you can do it for half an hour. Remember to check your pulse, and don't overdo it.

Biking.

One of the best activities for your heart, lower body muscles and weight loss, biking can be done in public on the streets or at home in the privacy of your bedroom. Pedaling faster, riding uphill, riding against the wind or pumping against greater resistance on a stationary bike burns extra energy.

Go at your own pace, gradually increasing the level of exertion. Remember to check your pulse rate periodically. Your pedaling should be done continuously and with some effort—coasting doesn't count!

Stepping.

If you want to exercise in private, this one's for you. You will need a step or a stool about seven inches high. Step up onto the step or stool with one foot; bring the other up beside it. Now step down with one foot; bring the other down, too. That's all there is to it, but it is one of the most strenuous exercises you can do because you are continuously lifting your entire body weight. So go slowly, and if you are very heavy or out of condition, wait until you have mastered the less strenuous forms of exercise. After warming up, do only four or five step-ups the first day, and slowly increase the number until you can keep it up for twenty minutes or half an hour without undue stress.

Stair Climbing.

This is the same idea as stepping, but you walk up and down stairs to achieve the same result. Because it is very demanding physically, monitor yourself, and stop immediately if you feel breathless or dizzy. Don't do it if you are extremely overweight. Remember to check your pulse periodically.

Here's what you do: After your warm-ups, walk up and down a flight of stairs, working up to half an hour, simple as that. Climb steadily and rhythmically, and if you need a rest between flights, walk up and down the hall for a minute or two.

(Stair climbing burns so much energy that researchers say you can lose ten to twelve pounds a year just by climbing an extra two flights of stairs a day.)

Avoid Reducing Suits

Never, never wear an exercise suit made of rubber or plastic, a so-called reducing suit. This can be extremely dangerous because it holds heat and does not allow the body's natural cooling system to function properly. It can lead to heat stroke.

SPECIAL SECTION FOR THE VERY OVERWEIGHT

If you are seriously overweight, you must be very cautious and careful about exercise, and be sure to be checked out by a physician before beginning any activity program. Remember to be patient, not to push yourself too much at first and to progress gradually through a well-planned program. And don't be tempted to try any of the activities on the "what not to do" list (page 230).

Here, direct from consultant Hyland Levasseur, physical fitness expert, is a special plan for you. First, a few important pointers:

1. Think of positive things as you work out, such as the fact that your body will continue to burn calories at a higher rate for several hours after you stop because the exercise raises your metabolism.

2. Start with "sittercises" and a five-minute nonstop walk every day; then progress according to the plan that follows. When you walk, don't worry about how fast you go, and don't exceed the prescribed time limit. It's a start in the right direction with minimum risk of injury or overexertion.

3. In the first three weeks or so of an exercise program, you may not lose weight, and you will certainly get stiff muscles. Don't get discouraged. After a few weeks you'll begin to lose weight quickly.

4. Keep in mind that nothing worthwhile in life comes easy.

5. Schedule at least five activity sessions per week. If you miss one, pick up your regular program at the next opportunity, always trying to maintain a minimum of three aerobic workouts each week. It's vital to take the time to exercise regularly if you want to lose a sufficient number of pounds.

How the Plan Works

· After about three months of sittercises and walking (Level 1), start doing your exercises while *standing,* and substitute exercycling for the walking. Or if you prefer, continue the walking instead, and try to step up your pace. This is Level 2.

· In another three months, advance to Level 3, taking your choice of swimming, walking or exercycling. Start at 220 yards (one-eighth mile) of nonstop swimming, using any style you want from dog paddle to backstroke, but keep moving. If swimming is out of the question for you, just continue your walking at a moderate pace, and increase the time by two minutes a week until you are up to thirty minutes of continuous walking at a moderate speed. A third choice: Continue exercycling at a slow pace, increasing the time by two minutes a week until you are doing thirty minutes nonstop.

· After working your way up to a half mile of continuous swimming, you may want to try rebounding (Level 4) if your doctor OKs it. First, you must acquire a rebounder, which is a mini-trampoline. Start jumping gently and jogging slowly on it for five minutes a day, following the progression outlined in Level 4. Or if rebounding doesn't appeal to you, though it's a different experience and fun for many people, continue swimming, walking or cycling.

· When you feel ready, decide if you want to start a walk-jog program. By now you should be thin enough to attempt it. Start at one mile total distance, walking and jogging intermittently, following the progression of Level 5. Or you may wish to continue walking or exercycling at the fifth level.

Sittercises
(Exercises Sitting in a Chair)

Start at three repetitions, and work up to ten repetitions for each exercise. Use a chair with no arms.

1. Seated Jumping Jacks

Swing arms overhead, touching the backs of your hands to each other, simultaneously moving your feet as far apart as possible. Return to starting position.

2. Hand Squeeze

Raise your arms straight out in front of you with the palms toward the floor. Open and close fists continuously without lowering your arms. Turn palms toward the ceiling, and repeat.

3. Arm Twists

Stretch your arms out to your sides with palms down. Now pull arms back as far as you can, and simultaneously turn palms toward the ceiling. Return to starting position.

4. Arm Circles

Stretch your arms out to your sides parallel to the floor with palms down. Make small circles forward, then small circles backward. Make large circles forward, then large circles backward.

5. Side Stretchers

Raise left hand overhead with palm toward the ceiling, place right hand on hip or arm of chair, lean to the right as far as possible and stretch four times. Now reverse the procedure, raising the right hand, placing the left on your hip, leaning to the left and stretching.

6. Wing Stretchers

Clench fists in front of chest with elbows out to the sides parallel to the floor. Pull elbows backward as far as you can, and return to starting position.

7. Arm Thrusts

Clench fists in front of chest with elbows out to the sides parallel to the floor. Thrust arms forward and back to the chest, to the side and back to the chest, upward and back to the chest, then down and back to the chest.

8. Reach for the Sky

Stretch both arms straight overhead as high as you can, at the same time spreading your fingers as wide as you can.

9. Overhead Stretch

Cup and clasp hands together, and extend them overhead. Now stretch up as far as you can.

10. Neck Benders

Bring head forward until chin touches your chest. Bring head backward as far as you can. Return to starting position. Turn head as far to the left as you can. Turn head as far to the right as you can. Return to starting position.

11. Toe Touches

Bend forward, reach down and touch your toes. Return to up-right position.

12. Single Leg Lifts

Sit up straight, and raise the right foot off the floor until your leg is completely straight. Lower slowly. Repeat with left leg.

13. Shoulder Shrugs

Rotate shoulders well up into the neck in a forward motion. Repeat in a reverse motion. Repeat in a straight up and down motion.

14. Deep Breathing

Inhale deeply through your nose, simultaneously lifting your arms overhead. Exhale slowly through your mouth as you bring your arms down.

Level 1

A. Sittercises. Every other day.

PLUS

B. Walking.   · Walk slowly for five minutes every other day.

· Add one minute every week until you are walking fifteen minutes nonstop.

Continue this program for about three months.

Level 2

A. Standing calisthenics. Do the same exercises you did sitting down, but exclude jumping jacks and single leg lifts. Do them every other day.

PLUS

B. Exercycling.   · Start at five minutes every other day at a slow pace.

· Add one minute every week up to fifteen minutes nonstop.

OR

Walking.   · Walk five minutes every other day at a moderate pace.

· Add one minute per week up to fifteen minutes nonstop.

Continue this program for about three months.

Level 3

A. Standing calisthenics. Every day.

PLUS

B. Swimming.   · Start at 220 yards (one-eighth mile) every other day. Add 55 yards every week up to a half mile of nonstop swimming.

OR

Walking.   · Walk fifteen minutes at a moderate pace. Add two minutes per week up to thirty minutes.

OR

Exercycling.   · Cycle fifteen minutes at a slow pace. Add two minutes a week up to thirty minutes.

Continue this program for about three months.

Level 4

A. Standing calisthenics. Every day.

PLUS

B. Rebounding.   · Start at five minutes slowly every day.
· Add one minute per week up to fifteen minutes.

OR

Walking.   · Walk twenty-five minutes at a moderate pace, then five minutes at a brisk pace.
· Add two minutes' brisk walking per week up to thirty minutes' continuous brisk walking.

OR

Exercycling.   · Exercycle for twenty-five minutes at a slow pace and five minutes at a moderate pace.
· Add two minutes per week up to thirty minutes.

Continue this program for about three months.

Level 5

A. Standing calisthenics, plus twenty-five sit-ups and ten modified push-ups every day.

PLUS

B. Walking-Jogging.   · Start at one mile, alternately walking and jogging as you like every day.
· When you can jog three-quarters of a mile nonstop, increase your total distance to one and a quarter miles.
· When you can jog one mile non-stop, increase total distance to one and a half miles.
· When you can jog one and a half miles nonstop, increase your total distance to one and three-quarters miles.
· Continue these progressions until you can jog two miles nonstop.

	OR
Walking.	· Walk at a brisk pace for thirty minutes.
	· Add two minutes at a brisk pace per week up to sixty minutes.
	OR
Exercycling.	· Exercycle for twenty-five minutes at a moderate pace, then five minutes at a brisk pace.
	· Add two minutes brisk-pace exercycling per week, up to thirty minutes continuous brisk-pace.

Exercises Not to Do If You Are Extremely Overweight

1. Jogging.

You can eventually jog if you follow the program given here, because you will have lost considerable weight before you reach Level 5. But before then jogging can be dangerous because of the extreme stress on the heart and legs.

2. Rope Jumping.

This, too, places great stress on the joints of the feet, ankles, knees and hips.

3. Weight Lifting.

Building muscle tissue which increases your weight, increasing your appetite and often causing dangerous increases in blood pressure, weight lifting is definitely not recommended.

4. Climbing Stairs.

Because stair climbing is very strenuous for a very overweight person, it should be avoided.

5. One-legged Exercises.

Any exercise that requires standing on one leg is dangerous because of the risk of losing your balance.

6. Competitive Sports.

Even at low levels, the sudden moves required may cause injury in a very overweight person who is not in condition.

Now you are on your way to success, perhaps for the first time in your overweight life. This time, by applying the methods developed at our renowned clinic at the Johns Hopkins, you will know how to get thin and stay that way.

The program doesn't promise miracles, but it promises results. If you stay with it, you will lose weight gradually and safely. And you can keep it off indefinitely. This is the proven route to significant weight loss, the antithesis of the quickie fad diets that don't work over the long term, based on our many years of research and experience.

Our program at Johns Hopkins, recently listed among only seven others by *Harper's Bazaar* as the best in the entire United States, really works. We have proved it. Thousands of people who never before managed to lose weight successfully have done it. You can too.

Index